D0390603

Walking in Divine Health

Walking in Divine Health

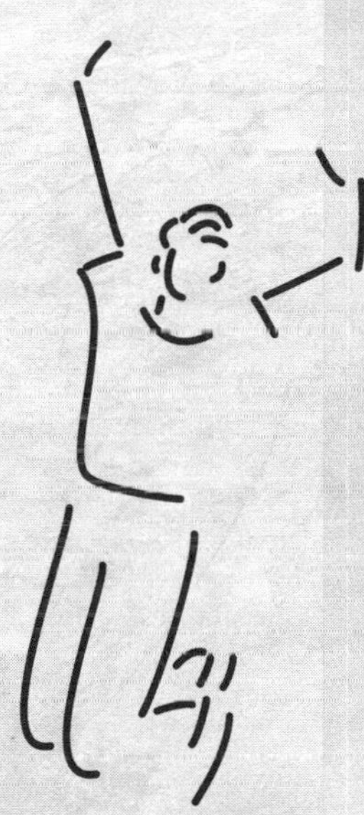

Don Colbert, M.D.

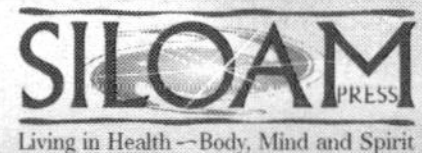

WALKING IN DIVINE HEALTH by Don Colbert, M.D.
Published by Siloam Press
A part of Strang Communications Company
600 Rinehart Road
Lake Mary, Florida 32746
www.siloampress.com

This book or parts thereof may not be reproduced in any form, stored in a retrieval system or transmitted in any form by any means–electronic, mechanical, photocopy, recording or otherwise–without prior written permission of the publisher, except as provided by United States of America copyright law.

Unless otherwise noted, all Scripture quotations are from the King James Version of the Bible.

Copyright © 1999 by Don Colbert, M.D.
All rights reserved

Interior design and typography by Terry Clifton

Library of Congress Cataloging-in-Publication Data:
Colbert, Don.
Walking in divine health / Don Colbert.
p. cm.
ISBN: 0-88419-626-7
1. Health–Religious aspects–Handbooks, manuals, etc.
2. Medicine in the Bible–Handbooks, manuals, etc.
3. Christian life–Handbooks, manuals, etc. I. Title
RA776.5.C635 1998
613–dc21 99-18239
CIP

Previously published by
Benny Hinn Media Ministries, copyright © 1996.
ISBN: 1-88125-93-5

This book is not intended to take the place of medical advice and treatment from your personal physician. Readers are advised to consult their own doctor or other qualified health professional regarding the treatment of their medical problems. Neither the publisher nor the author takes any responsibility for any possible consequences from any treament, action or application of medicine supplement, herb or preparation to any person reading or following the information in this book.

02 03 04 05 12 11 10 9 8
Printed in the United States of America

Dedication

To my son, Kyle, and to his generation, that they will learn from our mistakes and learn to walk in true divine health.

3 Eating to Live 103

4 *Finding Your Way Through the Vitamin and Supplement Maze* 139

Healing and Divine Health

HEALING AND DIVINE HEALTH ARE God's perfect will for mankind. God created Adam as a healthy being—a perfect act of creation. We find no record of sickness until Adam chose to disobey God. Sickness and disease entered the human race because of Adam's sin.

God's plan for man was that he would enjoy

divine health. The nature of our very makeup, beginning with the structure of each cell, supports this fact. Healing is constantly taking place in the human body. For example, what happens if you cut your finger? Regardless of the severity or size of the cut, the moment it occurs, every cell in your body begins to work in harmony to bring healing to that wound. Even the tiniest paper cut sets this healing process in motion, and in a matter of days the cut disappears, all because of the body's God-given ability to heal itself.

When considering the topic of health and healing, it is important to recognize that healing takes place in two realms: the natural and the divine. It's imperative that we understand how these two work together.

The Natural Realm

In the natural realm, a number of things contribute to the healing process. Included are medicines, doctors, exercise, good nutrition, proper amounts of sleep and the general good care of one's physical body. Doctors are God's servants, whether they know it or not. Even a doctor has to admit to a "higher power," or whatever name he uses to indicate God Almighty. The doctor can help you surgically, but only God can cause the incision made by the surgeon to heal.

God expects us to care for the physical bodies with which He has blessed us and not neglect or abuse them in any way. Several years ago I had an experience that helped me understand this principle of how the natural and divine realms work together. During the 1980s I began experiencing some occasional irregularities in my heartbeat. This condition affected me physically, and every now and then my heart would seem to miss a beat. When that occurred, I was forced to stop whatever I was doing and catch my breath.

As this condition continued, I became increasingly concerned about why God had not healed me. It became so severe that my doctor prescribed medication to slow down my heart rate. This was very difficult for me. Although I was involved in a healing ministry, I was forced to take a pill every day. As you might well imagine, it just didn't make sense to me.

In prayer, I complained to God about the situation. In total frustration I said, "Lord, I've prayed and I've prayed and I've prayed, and You have not healed me!"

To my surprise the Lord rebuked me and said, "Don't blame Me for what is your own fault." I was shocked! I can still remember thinking, *My own fault? What have I done wrong?*

I soon came to realize that I was neglecting to do what was right. I had not taken proper care of my body, and my ongoing neglect began to manifest itself through physical symptoms. Remember, faith begins where natural ability stops. I began an exercise program and started eating correctly. As I continued to modify my behavior, I noticed that my heart problem was less noticeable. Before long, it vanished completely.

This event underscored for me the two realms of healing–the natural and the divine. You must never ignore the natural realm. Exodus 15:26 declares:

> If thou wilt diligently hearken to the voice of the LORD thy God, and wilt do that which is right in his sight, and wilt

> give ear to his commandments, and keep all his statutes, I will put none of these diseases upon thee, which I have brought upon the Egyptians: for I am the LORD that healeth thee.

This is one of the many promises of healing contained in God's Word. Notice that it is in the present tense, for this is very important. God did not say, "I *was* the Lord who healed you," or "I *will be* the Lord who will heal you." He said, "I *am*," which implies He is continuously, forever our Healer. This promise is also conditional, for it begins with the word *if.* What does God mean by "if thou . . . wilt give ear to [My] commandments"? In my opinion, this means that we must give our best effort to live right. We can't live incorrectly and expect God to heal us. This is a covenant promise intended for those who live their lives according to God's guidelines. When we meet the conditions, the promise is ours. What God spoke two thousand years ago, He continues to say today.

I once heard a story about a lady who received a miracle of healing at an Aimee Semple McPherson meeting. Several months later, because she had become sick again, she attended another meeting that Aimee Semple McPherson was holding. She stood face to face with Aimee at one point and scolded her, saying, "Well, I thought I was healed!"

In response to the pointed remark, Aimee asked her what she had done after receiving her healing. Aimee was surprised to discover that the woman had gone back to the same habits and behaviors that had been so destructive to her body previously. After listening to the woman, Aimee stated emphatically, "Then it's your fault. Don't expect to stay healed if you're not going to do what is right."

God will heal you of incurable, debilitating diseases such as lung cancer, cirrhosis of the liver and the like. I've heard many glorious testimonies of such miracles. But when God touches a life miraculously, that individual must not return to the bad habits that may have caused the problem in the first place. We must understand that the natural realm exists; we cannot ignore it. If abusing your body produced a sickness, you must be willing to change your lifestyle–with God's help.

Healing is promised in the Bible, and God can

and will restore our health by taking away our sickness and disabilities. His will for us, however, as outlined in Scripture, is that we live in divine health, a state that is far better than divine healing. Scripture declares:

> Beloved, I wish above all things that thou mayest prosper and be in health, even as thy soul prospereth.
>
> –3 JOHN 2

In other words, God would prefer that we not get sick in the first place. That's what the Bible says. It is God's desire for His people to be healthy and prosperous, as 3 John 2 states. Unfortunately, many people today are sick, and this should not be so.

In our technologically advanced world, we are forced to breathe polluted air, drink treated water and eat chemically preserved foods. Nevertheless, the Bible says:

> And ye shall serve the LORD your God, and he shall bless thy bread, and thy water; and I will take sickness away from the midst of thee.
>
> –EXODUS 23:25

One day God said to me, "I'll protect you when it's impossible for you to know what you are taking into your body. But when you know, you are responsible."

I am very careful about what I eat. I feel that it is important to eat the right foods; in my opinion, healthy, nourishing foods are important to maintaining a healthy body. It's up to each one of us to choose a healthy lifestyle. Our bodies are our business. The Bible teaches that each one of us has a free will, and we are responsible for each decision we make. That means it is up to each individual to make good, healthy lifestyle choices.

The Divine Realm

It is possible to make all the right lifestyle choices and still get sick because of the limitations of the natural realm. It is also possible for an individual who has become ill to discover that the natural realm may not offer adequate help for regaining his or her health. When we have exhausted the natural realm, then we enter into the divine realm and trust the Lord. This is where the divine realm takes over, and God does what we cannot do.

The divine realm requires faith. It's in the divine realm that we appropriate the promises of God. Many have gone beyond the limitations of the natural realm, just as the woman did who had the issue of blood, as recorded in Mark 5. Scripture tells us that she had spent all of her money on physicians. Her condition, however, had not improved, and she had become worse. After she had pursued all the options that the natural realm offered, she sought help in the divine realm. In desperation she said, "If I may but touch the hem of His garment, I shall be made whole." When she reached out to touch the hem of Jesus' garment, she reached into the divine realm. The moment she reached out to Jesus, the Bible says:

> And straightway the fountain of her blood was dried up; and she felt in her body that she was healed of that plague.
>
> –MARK 5:29

She exercised her faith, and she was not disappointed.

Jesus testified of her healing:

> And he said unto her, Daughter, thy faith hath made thee whole; go in peace, and be whole of thy plague.
>
> –Mark 9:34

On many occasions I have made the following statement: Miracles begin where abilities cease. The woman with the issue of blood had exhausted every option in the natural realm and found that nothing cured her condition. She had spent everything she had and still had found no help. I have met so many individuals who never realized how priceless their health was until they lost it. And, like the woman with the issue of blood, they were willing to pay anything to regain it. But when the natural realm offered no help and with nowhere else to turn, they turned to Jesus and the divine realm. And as they reached out to the Master in faith, they were made whole by the healing power of God.

The woman with the issue of blood tried to touch the hem of His garment. It was not the touch of a hand that brought healing–it was the touch of faith. When the woman touched the hem of the Lord's garment, He felt virtue go out of Him and said, "Who touched Me?" Peter said, "Lord, many are touching You." There were many hands touching Jesus in the natural, but only one woman touched Him in faith.

If doctors have said, "We're sorry–there's no hope; there's nothing we can do for you," don't give up. God's Word promises, "I am the Lord that healeth thee." Reach out with your faith and touch Jesus.

When you do, your miracle will happen!

–Benny Hinn

Live in Health

PICTURE A MERCEDES BENZ OR A BMW; both are incredible pieces of machinery. What would happen to either of these automobiles if you did not change the oil regularly? What if you put water in your Mercedes's gas tank instead of gasoline? What if you never had it serviced, failed to put air in the tires and never replaced the air filter? Instead, you simply drove it constantly and recklessly. What if you left road salts and acids on the body and frame? What would be the life span of this expensive automobile?

Millions of individuals are doing the same thing to their bodies. We're filling our tanks with junk foods and wondering, *Why do I always feel so exhausted?* We're subjecting our bodies to environmental toxins and wondering why we contract diseases.

Friend, on these pages I will tell you how you can live in health and have tremendous energy every day of your life. Through years of research and study, volumes and volumes have been written on the process of disease. Although it is often difficult to make complex information simple, I have attempted to assemble a handbook of information based upon biblical principles to help believers walk in divine health.

As a medical doctor, I am deeply troubled as I see younger and younger people stricken with cancer, heart disease and many other diseases. Millions of people are caught up in a fast-paced, fast-food lifestyle that has little regard for health and nutrition. I believe God has the power to heal, and I have personally witnessed many miracles that only He could have performed. I also believe that He desires that His people live healthy lives by obeying principles of good health that are as old as creation. Interspersed throughout this book, you will find thirty-four healthy living tips.

It is my prayer that the material in this book will equip you with the knowledge to walk in divine health, enabling you to better serve our Creator and Lord.

While I am excited about presenting this material to you, as a medical doctor I understand the importance of discussing any changes you plan to make regarding diet, prescriptions or lifestyle with your physician.

–Don Colbert, M.D.

Chapter 1

Stopping Cancer Before It Starts

An incident occurred on Friday, April 26, 1986, at 1:23 A.M. that significantly impacted our world. It was not reported that day on the local evening news; neither was it carried by any worldwide news distribution agency.

The event: an explosion in a nuclear reactor in the Chernobyl nuclear plant, located near Kiev in

Ukraine. Although the magnitude of the blast blew the roof off the reactor, spewing fifty tons of radioactive fuel into the sky and forming a huge cloud of radiation gases, it was neither immediately discovered nor disclosed.

Three days later, hundreds of miles away in Sweden, an employee at a Swedish nuclear power plant reported for work as usual. When he entered the nuclear power plant through the standard screening area, loud bells, whistles and alarms began sounding, indicating an abnormal level of radiation. He was immediately checked, and to the surprise of everyone, high doses of radiation were found on the soles of his shoes.

Additional testing revealed that the air over Sweden contained more than one hundred times the normal level of radiation. The huge cloud of radioactive gases that had formed in the air over Chernobyl three days earlier was not detected until it drifted over Sweden. Research finally determined the original source and uncovered the nuclear disaster that had occurred at Chernobyl.

The entire incident, along with the huge cloud of radiation gases in the air, had not been reported.

As time passed, the radiation continued to move over Europe. As it drifted on its way, it poisoned the water, the rivers, the animals and ultimately the food chain.

What impact did the Chernobyl incident have upon our world, and what will be the future consequences? Is this crisis over, or has it just begun?

Living Healthy Tip No. 1

Cruciferous vegetables, which include broccoli, cabbage, cauliflower, collards and mustard greens, contain powerful phytochemicals that protect us from esophageal, stomach, colon, prostate and breast cancer.

As a medical doctor I am disheartened to see the incidence of cancer increasing in our society. Current statistics indicate that one out of every three people will develop some form of cancer in his or her lifetime. I believe that between 80 and 90 percent of cancers can be prevented because they are caused by environmental, dietary or nutritional factors.

Every year, billions of dollars are spent on cancer treatment and research. Yet with all we have invested in cancer during this century, the death rate caused by this disease continues to climb. It is a sobering fact.

Three main types of cancer are most commonly diagnosed in the United States:

- Lung cancer
- Colon and rectal cancer
- Breast cancer

Combined, these three are responsible for approximately 50 percent of all cancer deaths in our nation annually.

Lung Cancer

We don't stop to realize it, but when someone lights up a cigarette, more than two thousand chemicals are released in that smoke. Even more alarming is the fact that most hazardous chemicals come from the lighted end–which is the source of secondhand smoke (the passive smoke we all inhale).

You may never have smoked in your life, but you are inhaling danger when you are near someone who is smoking. Whether in restaurants, at the ball park or in the lobby of a concert hall, you are consuming secondhand toxins.

In 1986 the U.S. Surgeon General determined that passive smoke was definitely associated with lung cancer–the most deadly form of cancer known today. Here is what happens: The smoke coming from cigarettes produces harmful free radicals that change the DNA–the genetic material in your cells. A *free radical*, according to Webster's dictionary, is an atom or a group of atoms having at least one unpaired electron and participating in various reactions. The smoke changes the DNA in your cells to a different DNA, which begins growing like wildfire when it's exposed to other environmental promoters.

Colon Cancer

Why do we have so much cancer of the colon in our society? It is because the foods we eat contain toxins that stay in our gastrointestinal tracts for days simply because we don't eat enough fiber in our foods. Because of the lack of sufficient fiber to help with elimination, toxins remain in our gastrointestinal tracts and begin to form carcinogens. Eventually these carcinogens begin to change the cells of the colon. In my medical practice I diagnose abnormal polyps, or precancerous growths, regularly.

Colon cancer, the second leading cause of cancer death, is at epidemic proportions in our country because of two reasons:

- The percentage of pesticides and toxins we are taking into our bodies
- The low fiber content of the foods we eat

The solution lies in eating fruits and vegetables that contain enough fiber to help bind toxins and eliminate them from the colon.

The often-used phrase "you are what you eat" is true. Consequently, if we consume large amounts of toxins on a continuous basis–whether knowingly or unknowingly–we will be affected.

Most people go through life unaware they are ingesting toxins. They are taking in industrial toxins, pesticides and many kinds of harmful fat. Foods containing such substances go through our digestive tracts and actually transform cells into carcinogenic cells, which eventually become the polyps that form cancer.

Fortunately, colon cancer is more frequently diagnosed than any other terminal form of cancer, and many cases are successfully treated as a result. Although skin cancer is diagnosed more frequently than colon cancer, it is not considered a terminal form of cancer because people seldom die from it. Colon cancers, on the other hand, are killers. They are also associated with a high intake of red meat and animal fat, high cholesterol, low fiber and obesity.

Most Americans take in far too little fiber. The lowest incidences of colon cancer are found in Third World countries such as Africa, Asia and South America. Why? Because these people eat more fiber and less fat. Their diets consist of vegetables, fruits and grains–high fiber foods that are the key to their low rates of cancer.

Breast Cancer

The most common type of cancer in women is breast cancer. According to current statistics, one in eight women will develop breast cancer. It used to be one in ten, but breast cancer is on the rise.

Why is this the case? The major contributing factors are the toxins and pesticides that we take into our bodies. These substances are stored in the fatty tissues of animals. Women ingest these toxins through the meat and food they eat, and the toxins are then stored in the fattiest portion of a woman's body: the breast.

For women, breast cancer is the second-leading cause of cancer deaths in the United States. The first is lung cancer. Breast cancer is linked to high levels of consumption of animal fats and whole milk products. From early childhood we are told, "Drink milk; it's good for you." Now we know that if we drink milk, it should not be whole milk but skim milk or milk products with greatly reduced fat content.

We should also select cheeses made with skim milk instead of those produced with whole milk. I tell my patients not to eat butter or ice cream because these foods contain the hormone estrogen from cows. Dairy cows are injected with DES, which is a form of estrogen. Small amounts of this hormone, when taken into the body, can be found in women's breasts. Whole milk products also contain fat and cholesterol, which provide the raw materials for making additional estrogen. Your body will make more estrogen using the actual fat that contains pesticides and other carcinogens. This is how toxins find their home in the fatty tissues in the breast.

Prostate cancer is occurring in epidemic proportions as is breast cancer, and for the same reasons. The prostate is a fatty gland, and toxins, as I mentioned, are stored in fatty tissues.

Living Healthy Tip No. 2

Soy foods—including tofu, soy milk, soy meat substitutes, soy flour, soy protein flour and roasted soy nuts—contain phytochemicals and reduce the risk of breast, colon, lung and stomach cancer.

Understanding the Facts

Sadly, because of the foods we eat, it is commonly known that the world's highest incidences of cancer are concentrated in the United States.

Approximately 97 percent of the cells in your

body are replaced every year from the nutrients that you take in. What you ingest actually becomes a part of the structure of your body. That's why proper nutrition is so important.

Free Radicals

It is vital to learn about free radicals, since they are essential in understanding cancer–how it starts and how we can protect ourselves from it.

First, we need to understand the process of oxidation, which is a chemical procedure. For example, when metals are oxidized, rust is produced. When oxidation occurs on painted surfaces, the paint begins to flake off. When you cut an apple in half, it turns brown–that is oxidation. It also occurs when meat rots. Our bodies are undergoing oxidative processes every day, and we need to know how to protect ourselves from free radicals and oxidation.

Oxidation is actually caused by free radicals. What happens when you place lemon juice on an exposed slice of an apple? The apple slice doesn't turn brown because the lemon blocks the oxidative process–it stops the formation of free radicals.

For a moment, picture an atom. It has a nucleus, and it has electrons around it. The nucleus is positively charged, and the electrons are negatively charged. It would look something like the sun with the planets around it.

What happens when someone blows smoke in your face or you are exposed to air pollution or radiation? Or what happens when you take in alcohol or some other chemical or pesticide? High energy radiation in the air pollution, or chemicals in the smoke, will knock electrons out of orbit. This can create free radicals that affect living tissue. This energy in radiation grabs one of the electrons out of orbit, and suddenly power is transferred over to that electron, which then seeks another atom, moving into that atom's orbit. That atom then becomes an unstable atom, and a chain reaction has begun–one to the other, and then to the next–caused by those free radicals.

A similar process involving free radicals is associated with the formation of many cancers. Fortunately God has placed within our grasp a solution to the problem of free radicals. It is available in the form of antioxidants, which we will soon discuss. Since our bodies are constantly renewed and replaced by the nutrients we take in, this issue is critically important. We must act to help our cells prevent degenerative diseases.

How Does Cancer Develop?

The first step on the path that leads to cancer is taken by an "initiator." An example of this process is found in the act of smoking cigarettes. When a person smokes, the cancer-causing process actually starts with the tobacco. But the cancer doesn't start fueling or spreading until it has a "promoter." A promoter is a substance that enables the initiated cell to take off and start growing abnormally.

Another example of a promoter is estrogen. Giving a woman estrogen who still has her uterus and is not being given progesterone (which is another female hormone) with it can begin the cancer promotion process in the uterus.

Another illustration is a man with prostate cancer. If that man were prescribed testosterone, the cancer could be fueled. Other known promoters of cancer are polyunsaturated fats, saturated fats, red meats and foods high in cholesterol.

Why do vegetarians have a much lower incidence of cancer? It is because they eat 25 percent less fat and 50 percent more fiber. This gives them added protection.

The Japanese people have a very low incidence of cancer when they reside in Japan, but when they come to the United States and take up our dietary practices, such as eating at fast-food establishments, they develop essentially the same incidence of cancer as we have. The message is clear. We live and die because of the food we place in our bodies. It is imperative that we become more disciplined and make the right dietary choices.[1]

Living Healthy Tip No. 3

Tomatoes contain lycopene, which is a potent phytochemical that will reduce the risk of developing colon and prostate cancer.

I believe in medicine, but I also believe in prayer. Before you begin to eat your food, pause for a moment, not only to thank God for it, but to pray over it in faith. We must act in faith every time we eat because of all the pesticides and carcinogens to which we are exposed on a daily basis.

Antioxidants

An antioxidant is a vitamin, a mineral, an enzyme, a phytonutrient (a plant nutrient) or a food. Antioxidants have the ability to bind free radicals and to neutralize them. In reality, an antioxidant pairs up that electron and stops that dangerous chain reaction of events.

We've had antioxidants for years, but now we've got super antioxidants that everyone should know about and most people should be taking.

An antioxidant with which many people are familiar is vitamin E. This antioxidant works to prevent free radical damage that can cause cancer or heart disease. By taking vitamin E we are helping to protect ourselves from these dreaded diseases.

Where do you find vitamin E? In nuts, seeds, whole grains and also in polyunsaturated fats. However, we should not eat polyunsaturated fats such as canola oil or corn oil, since they can cause the formation of additional free radicals.

The oil you should take into your body is extra virgin olive oil. We need to avoid saturated fats and polyunsaturated fats but welcome monounsaturated fats. These are the good fats that are found in olive oil and are very protective. A word of caution: Don't rush out and consume tons of olive oil, or you'll end up weighing 300 pounds! Nonetheless, when you see a recipe that calls for oil, use olive oil.

The RDA (recommended daily allowance) for vitamin E is only 15 International Units a day. That is not going to give you much protection. I take 800 units a day. I recommend that you take more than the RDA amount–between 400 and 800 units a day for protection. In addition, when purchasing vitamin E, choose the natural form and not the synthetic form.

Vitamin C

If you are like most people, when you think of vitamin C you probably think of orange juice.

However, there are many other foods with this important vitamin, including broccoli, peppers, turnip greens, collard greens and parsley.

A plant grown commonly in West India called acerola is very high in vitamin C. One glass of orange juice (3½ ounces) contains only 50 milligrams of vitamin C, whereas 3½ ounces of acerola has 1,300 milligrams.

Linus Pauling, a Nobel Prize winner, was recognized as one of the greatest researchers ever. He recommends between 1 to 10 grams (1,000 to 10,000 milligrams) of vitamin C every day. The recommended daily allowance of vitamin C is only 60 milligrams a day. Pauling lived until his mid-nineties, much longer than the average life span of a doctor. He credited his longevity to the high doses of vitamin C.[2]

Living Healthy Tip No. 4

Garlic has antibiotic, antiviral and antifungal ingredients. It will decrease the risk of developing stomach cancer.

I take 1,000 milligrams of vitamin C three times a day. If you're in a period of stress or illness, you could take even more–perhaps one and a half times that amount. It is very inexpensive. Vitamin C is critically important; you may want to begin by taking 2,000 milligrams (2 grams) a day, taken in two 1,000-milligram doses.

Vitamin A

Foods that are considered high sources of vitamin A include liver, kidneys, butter and whole milk. As you can imagine, I would not recommend eating liver or kidney since these organs are filters where toxins are stored. And since we should avoid eating butter and drinking whole milk, we should forget about getting vitamin A from our foods. Instead we should get it from beta carotene, which is similar but not the same thing.

Beta carotene is pro–vitamin A, and your body can make all the vitamin A it needs from beta carotene without becoming toxic. Because you can become toxic by taking vitamin A, I don't recommend taking vitamin A supplements. I tell my patients to take beta carotene, which is found in dark green leafy vegetables such as spinach and collards. Spinach can be high in pesticide residues, so you might want to purchase organically grown spinach or wash it extremely well. Other sources of beta carotene are carrots, sweet potatoes, yams, squash and other yellow or orange vegetables.

Consider buying a juicer to provide an alternate way to take in greater amounts of nutrients from the natural sources of fruits and vegetables without actually eating the entire products. For example, I recommend carrot juice to any of my patients who have cancer since it is rich in beta carotene.

If you prepare carrot juice you must drink it immediately. If you let it stand after juicing it will lose its potency. This is also true with vitamin C. If you don't eat fruits promptly, they lose their antioxidant effect.

Vitamin A, beta carotene, vitamin E and vitamin C are the major antioxidant vitamins. You can get them in an over-the-counter supplement. However, don't expect to get a high dosage from a multivitamin. You may have to buy an antioxidant formula or purchase each vitamin individually.

Antioxidant vitamins are important, and you

need to get those that are natural and have a nice gelatin coating or a coating that dissolves easily. You can test a vitamin's coating by seeing how quickly it dissolves in vinegar.

Minerals

Some potent antioxidants are found in minerals. Three in particular are outstanding: zinc, copper and manganese.

Our soils have been called mineral depleted, and for an unusual reason. In the 1940s the large companies that produced nitrates and phosphates for ammunition during World War II had to switch over to producing something else because they could no longer use the nitrates and the phosphates for ammunition. They began to make fertilizer from a combination of nitrogen, phosphorus and potassium. Such fertilizer produced incredibly beautiful crops.

Prior to this time, farmers used crop rotation, mowing and mulching to keep soils from losing precious minerals. Following the war, companies began to place these chemicals into very inexpensive fertilizers. With the use of these fertilizers, crop rotation became unnecessary. The farmers seemed to have no choice. If they continued rotating their crops and did not use the fertilizers, they would go out of business because of the increased productivity of their neighbors who were using the new products.

Consequently, over the years we depleted our soil of some very important minerals. Because of what has happened to our soil, our crops no longer supply us with the minerals we need.

Nitrogen, phosphorus and potassium provide three main minerals in fertilizer, but we need twenty-two essential minerals for optimal health, and at least fifty essential nutrients. If you're expecting to receive all your minerals from foods, it's highly unlikely that you will.

Zinc, copper and manganese form a very potent antioxidant called SOD, or superoxide dismutase. This enzyme is a very powerful antioxidant that actually neutralizes free radicals and prevents damage to our cell membranes. When the membranes are being assaulted by smoke, radiation from the sun, poisons or chemicals, SOD acts to repair them. If we don't have enough zinc, copper and manganese, the repair process will not be as effective.

The best way to receive these elements is through a process that is called chelated mincrals. Chelated minerals help to absorb zinc, copper and manganese. You can get zinc and copper through nuts and legumes such as beans and peas. Manganese is found in pecans, Brazil nuts, almonds and barley.

Living Healthy Tip No. 5

Take a complex multivitamin, mineral and antioxidant supplement daily to prevent micronutrient deficiencies that can lead to degenerative diseases.

Selenium

Selenium and glutathione make up another very important antioxidant called glutathione peroxidase. Selenium is a mineral that is found in meats and grains (depending on the soil content). It is also found in Brazil nuts, broccoli, garlic and onions.

Glutathione

Glutathione is made from cysteine, the amino acid that comes from eating protein. It protects cell membranes. Imagine a little cell being bombarded daily by free radicals. Each cell receives about ten thousand free radical hits to the DNA each day, according to some scientists. Glutathione simply scavenges and neutralizes the free radicals and restores and protects your cell membranes.

Coenzyme Q-10

Another antioxidant is coenzyme Q-10. Very few people know about it, but it is very potent. It's a vitamin-like substance, very similar to vitamin E and very essential. You find it in fish such as mackerel, Pacific salmon and sardines. Coenzyme Q-10 is a potent antioxidant and is very good for your immune system. It also scavenges free radicals and strengthens your cell membranes. It plays a major role in energy production. If your energy level is at an all-time low, coenzyme Q-10 will definitely help boost your energy level. It's important to supplement our diets with this antioxidant, because we don't get enough in our foods.

Super antioxidants

Super antioxidants will help you walk in health. One in particular is twenty times more powerful than vitamin C and fifty times more powerful than vitamin E. It is grape seed extract.

The French eat as much as Americans and smoke more cigarettes, but they have half the risk of heart disease as Americans. This is largely due to French people's consumption of red wine. Red grapes from colder climates, such as France and Canada, usually have a higher concentration of resveratrol. Resveratrol is the main phytonutrient in red wine, which protects from both heart disease and cancer. Taking one capsule of resveratrol twice daily is equivalent to drinking two glasses of nonalcoholic wine from France or Canada each day.

Contained within the seed of a grape is a

powerful antioxidant called a flavonoid (more than twenty thousand bioflavonoids exist). There are other flavonoids, such as pine bark extract that comes from the European coastal pine trees and is also an excellent antioxidant. But grape seeds are in a family by themselves. Research shows that grape seed extract is at the top of the list as the most active antioxidant of all.

Phytonutrients

A new group of chemicals are revolutionizing nutrition. In particular, phytonutrients (plant nutrients that are chemical extracts taken from plants) contain very effective antioxidants. They also contain enzyme simulators and have hormone inhibitors. Researchers are now using these substances to treat cancer patients.

Living Healthy Tip No. 6

Most Americans are already in the process of developing cancer due to their lack of exercise, stressful lifestyles and the amount of processed food, sugar, hydrogenated and polyunsaturated fats in their diets.

Do you remember the television characters called the Jetsons? They took little pills instead of food. The parents said, "Now take your carrots and have your broccoli," as they handed little orange and green pills to their children. Now science has isolated and extracted the most potent chemicals in our vegetables, and these chemicals can be extracted and shaped into pills. They work like a drug in preventing disease. In cancer patients, the results of early research at Harvard and other medical research centers have been phenomenal.

The protease inhibitor

Found in a plant's reproductive parts–especially in the soybean–is a substance called the protease inhibitor. This is actually the seed's defense against destruction. Birds can swallow the seed, but can't digest this substance. It is excreted. What is unique about a protease inhibitor is that it cannot be broken down.

This tiny part of the soybean seed can block

both the initiation and the promotion of certain cancers. That is why medical scientists are excited now about these plant chemicals. Some research has shown cells that have been reprogrammed back to their original precancerous state.

Flavonoids

There are many classes of flavonoids. These potent anticancer agents are found in green tea, soybeans, celery and cruciferous vegetables including cabbage, Brussels sprouts and broccoli.

Polyphenols

Another phytochemical is polyphenol. It is found in garlic, soybeans, green tea, cruciferous vegetables and umbelliferous vegetables such as carrots. Polyphenols are antioxidants that act to prohibit both the initiation and promotion of cancer–they either block it or they slow it down.

Polyphenols can also be found in the ellagic acid in strawberries and grapes. These tasty fruits are excellent for you, but get pesticide-free strawberries and grapes, or wash them with a fruit and vegetable rinse.

Sulfides

Sulfides are found in garlic and in cruciferous vegetables (such as cabbage and broccoli); they stimulate the repair of DNA. When you're exposed to smoke or carcinogens, DNA can be broken down and need restoration. The result of research on sulfides has been nothing short of amazing.

If you know anyone with cancer, or someone who has a strong family history of cancer, I recommend they begin to take these nutrients as soon as possible. Encourage him or her to begin juicing these vegetables.

Terpenes

Another important antioxidant is terpene. It is found in garlic, cruciferous vegetables and umbelliferous vegetables. This also helps to block the initiation and growth of cancer.

Phytoestrogen

Phytoestrogen, found in soy products, inhibits breast cancer by blocking the effects of estrogen. Women who have a family history of breast cancer should take this nutrient.

Two additional helpful anticancer agents are indoles and lycopenes. Indoles are plant sugars found in cabbage, broccoli, cauliflower, Brussels sprouts and radishes. They stimulate the protective enzymes that help to reduce the initiation of cancer. Lycopene is found in tomatoes and is a strong anticancer chemical. Presently, more than thirty phytonutrients are being investigated and developed–and there are many more to be discovered.

Incredible Vegetables and Fruits

Soybeans

There is a food that has been cultivated for thousands of years and is one of America's most important crops. It is the soybean, a vegetable that has been fed to our farm animals but not eaten, to a great extent, by humans. Yet it has been found to be one of the foods most effective in protecting us from cancer. Soybeans are used in the making of tofu, soy sauce, soy flour and soy milk.

Now that I understand its special properties, I tell everyone they need to be eating more soybeans in any form they can. Nutritionists say that one cup of soybeans is equivalent to one regular tablet of Premarin, which is a form of estrogen. This is important because it can help prevent breast cancer.

Living Healthy Tip No. 7

The most dangorous foods for cancer patients are those highest in sugar and hydrogenated fats, which include donuts and pastries.

Soybeans also have isoflavones, phytoestrogen and the protease inhibitors. Best of all, soy products help reduce the risk of lung, colon and breast cancer. In one research study, women regularly consuming soy foods had nearly 50 percent less cancer than those who did not.

Cruciferous vegetables

This category of vegetables is extremely important in stimulating the body to detoxify and eliminate cancer-causing chemicals. Cruciferous vegetables include cabbage, broccoli, cauliflower, Brussels sprouts, collard and mustard greens, turnip greens and radishes.

Cabbage in particular is one of the most important nutrient foods that you can eat. It has potent anticancer properties that help the body protect against the damage of free radicals. It also has polyphenols that act as garbage collectors, ridding the body of carcinogens. In addition, it has indoles, which stimulate protective enzymes that help protect us from cancer. The more cabbage we eat, the lower our risk of breast and colon cancer.

Coleslaw made with fat-free mayonnaise is a great addition to your daily diet. Eat it every day if possible.

Green tea

Green tea is a drink that decreases the risk of

cancer and is common in the Orient, but is much less common here in the United States. The tea leaves are not heated but are actually steamed, rolled and crushed. It's been a favorite in Japan for over a thousand years, and it is loaded with polyphenols. The antioxidant activity of green tea is two hundred times more potent than that of vitamin E and five hundred times more potent than vitamin C. To help prevent cancer, one should drink two to three cups of green tea each day.

Garlic

Garlic has been used in Egypt for more than five thousand years and in China for more than three thousand years. It was used to treat the great plague in Europe and as a cure for dysentery during World War I. Now we know that garlic has antifungal, antiviral and antibacterial properties. I take garlic every day in an odorless form.

Parsley

An important anticancer phytonutrient is

found in parsley. This nutrient also inhibits the cancer-causing properties of fried foods.

Tomatoes

The wonderful tomato is not only good to eat but contains three phytonutrients that help prevent the formation of carcinogens. Eat tomatoes regularly, sliced, in salads or as a juice. According to a Health Professionals Fellowship study of forty-seven thousand subjects, a man who eats ten servings of foods containing tomatoes each week will reduce his risk of developing prostate cancer by 45 percent.

Strawberries and grapes

Strawberries and grapes contain an important acid–ellagic acid–that neutralizes cancer and the toxins that cause cancer. They also protect against damage to our chromosomes.

Tangerines

The tangerine is filled with a strong phytonutrient called *tangeretin.* It inhibits the invasiveness of cancer. Research is also being conducted regarding its ability to help slow the spread of breast cancer. Try to eat tangerines as often as possible. They do not contain pesticides and are effective warriors against cancer.

Yogurt

Yogurt contains lactobacillus, acidophilus and bifidus bacteria–good bacteria that help combat carcinogens in our gastrointestinal tracts. These good bacteria help reduce the production of cancer-causing chemicals. Eat a small container of yogurt every day (not the high sugar, high-fat varieties) to help prevent cancer.

Enzymes

Enzymes are critical to health and essential in the digestion and assimilation of food. They protect our cells and are found in raw foods, but not in processed or most fast foods.

Many people who don't eat fresh fruits and vegetables regularly are deficient in enzymes. If you cook food at a temperature of over 118 degrees Fahrenheit, you destroy essential enzymes that manufacture strong cells we need to combat disease and illness.

Eating enzyme-deficient foods may mean that our foods are not absorbed properly or used and converted to energy.

We are born with a limited ability to make enzymes, and we must either get them from the food we eat or from a supplement. The best advice is to eat raw foods—not cooked or steamed. Food in its fresh, raw state has all its enzymes; those enzymes help us to digest the raw foods and release the nutrients in them that our bodies need.

Living Healthy Tip No. 8

Cancer is increasing at such an alarming rate that about 40 percent of Americans will develop cancer, but only 14 percent of Americans who exercise regularly will develop cancer.

To Sum It Up

To decrease your risk of cancer:

- Maintain your ideal body weight.
- Decrease your fat intake.
- Switch from eating fatty foods to lean meats such as chicken or turkey.
- Switch from using whole milk, whole milk cheeses, butter, cream and ice cream to low-fat skim milk and skim milk cheeses.
- Do not eat margarine. It contains trans-fatty acids that can contribute to heart disease.
- Avoid butter. It is full of fat and has unwanted chemicals. Use a substitute such as Butter Buds.
- Increase your fiber intake. Take in 25 to 30 grams of fiber a day.
- If you smoke, stop! You are killing yourself; worse yet, you're killing your loved ones.
- Do not drink alcohol. It is also associated with free radical damage and with cancer.

Take grape seed extract instead or drink nonalcoholic red wine.

- Remember the foods that contain nitrites and avoid them, such as luncheon meats (bologna and salami) and bacon.
- Avoid smoked meats, salt-cured meats and other high-pesticide foods.
- Take antioxidants such as vitamin C, vitamin E and beta carotene.
- Take minerals including selenium, zinc, copper and manganese.
- It's best to get minerals in chelated form. Most are found in a good multivitamin.
- Do not forget about coenzyme Q-10.
- Take an enzyme supplement before eating processed foods or overcooked vegetables in which the enzymes have been depleted.
- Eat plenty of fresh fruits and vegetables.
- If you have cancer or a strong family history of cancer, get phytonutrients that are found in carrots, broccoli and cabbage.

- Start eating soybeans and tofu and drinking green tea.
- Eat plenty of cruciferous vegetables.

If you do these simple things and exercise regularly, you will reduce your risk of cancer significantly and be well on your way to walking in divine health.

NOTES

WALKING IN DIVINE HEALTH

Walking in Divine Health

Walking in Divine Health

Walking in Divine Health

Chapter 2

Slamming the Door on Heart Disease

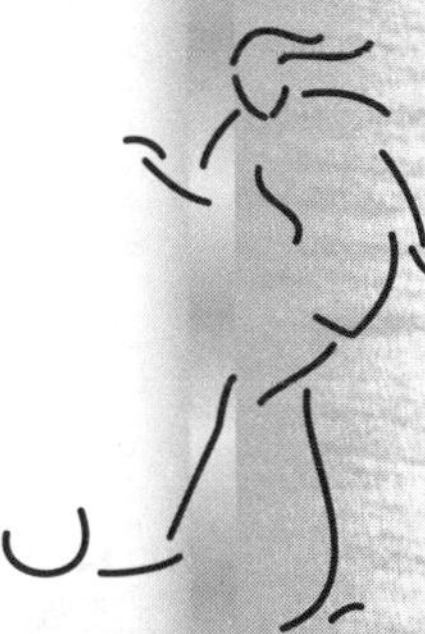

RECENTLY A LADY IN MY OFFICE TOLD ME that her father had passed away because of a massive heart attack. She explained that he was a successful businessman in his fifties. He had just bought a condominium and was celebrating with his attorney. Recalling the details, she said, "He was eating a big fat steak, a baked potato with lots of butter and drinking some alcohol. Later that evening he suffered a massive heart attack and died."

They wheeled the man into the emergency room and did a heart scan. A close friend of the patient came out to the waiting room in tears. "I cannot believe it. The attack has destroyed over 90 percent of his heart muscle."

When the heart muscle dies, there is little you can do. He was slated for a heart transplant but died before the procedure was possible.

Approximately 40 percent of people will develop a heart attack and not even have a symptom. If you're waiting for a signal, it will probably come too late. Don't think, *Well, when I start having a little chest pain, or when I start feeling something in my heart, then I'll change my behavior and lower my fat intake.* No, a heart attack is like a poisonous snake slithering toward you in the dark. It strikes when you least expect it.

You may ask, "How could one huge meal, even with all those fats, trigger an attack?" After a meal laden with heavy fats, your blood–all of it–becomes thicker than usual. One doctor described it as being "as thick as toothpaste."

Fats and oils in the blood increase its density. The heart has to pump blood that at times can resemble sludge. I've checked the blood of patients after they have eaten lunch, and it is amazing how much fat is present. It rises to the top of the venipuncture tube, and you can actually see it. It is yellow and thick. Just imagine what that fat is doing to your blood vessels when the heart is attempting to pump it through your system.

For many people there comes a time when their hearts are doing their best to push their blood through the vessels, and then suddenly it happens. BOOM! They grasp their chests and feel the terrifying pain of a heart attack.

Living Healthy Tip No. 9

Maintaining ideal body weight will dramatically decrease your chance of developing heart disease, diabetes and other degenerative diseases.

The fact that 60 percent of those who have an attack survive it should be of no comfort. It's not worth playing the odds. Can you be certain that you will not be among the other 40 percent?

Heart disease is deadly. And since it affects almost everyone directly or indirectly, it is imperative to know how to avoid it in our own lives, in the lives of our children, in the lives of our parents and in the lives of those we love.

This discussion may frighten some people, yet it needs to be dealt with without apology. Many people are dying early in life because they are not obeying God's dietary laws.

God's Dietary Laws

As believers we are here to serve the Lord, but many great men and women of God are not fulfilling His will because they fail to heed His commands. Here is a nutritional warning from the Bible:

> It shall be a perpetual statute for your generations throughout all your dwellings, that ye eat neither fat nor blood.
>
> –LEVITICUS 3:17

Do you know what "perpetual statute" suggests?

It was a law given not only for the moment, but for all ages of time. And what is the command? It is a severe warning that we should not eat fat or blood.

At the time this command was given, the people were not eating fat on their bread, or adding it to their foods, yet God gave the warning. Could it be that the blatant disregard of this passage of Scripture has resulted in the epidemic of heart disease across our land?

Today, one million Americans die each year of heart and blood vessel diseases. These diseases are responsible for one out of two deaths. Think of it–more people die of heart disease than are killed by cancer, infectious disease, AIDS, homicides and accidents combined. I'm convinced we are dying of coronary disease because of the fat we eat. Just look around and you will see the danger–fast-food restaurants are popping up everywhere.

Many of you will choose to ignore these pages because your craving for a diet containing fat is more than a habit; it's an addiction. The bottom line, however, is this: If you act on the information I am about to give you, it will mean life. If you ignore it, it can lead to disease and death.

I wish I could tell you there is a shortcut to good health, but I can't. You cannot take one pill, however powerful, and follow it with a huge meal of pork ribs, French fries and ice cream. The two will never balance, and you will continue your slide toward a future filled with illness and infirmity. Instead, you must begin with God's first nutritional law that says you shall not eat of the fat.

I realize how difficult it is to apply everything this book contains. But I want to give you the tools to accomplish at least one important goal–to greatly reduce your intake of this deadly killer.

The Sudden Attack

We have all heard the term *cardiovascular disease*, but exactly what does it mean? *Cardio* means "heart," and *vascular* means "blood vessel."

The word *arteriosclerosis* is similar. *Arterio* means "artery," and *sclerosis* means "hardening" or "scarring," usually from a buildup of cholesterol. A coronary, or heart attack, is most often the result of the coronary arteries, which supply the heart with blood, becoming clogged with plaque.

The heart is an organ about the size of your fist which beats day and night–at sixty to eighty beats a minute. Two main arteries encircle the heart and branch down and around it to supply this muscle with blood and oxygen. Our bodies are totally dependent upon a good supply of blood flowing through our arteries to nourish our hearts and send enough blood to keep them pumping continually. When you stop to think about it, it is amazing that the heart can keep going at its constant, steady pace.

The arteries are lined with a smooth lining called the *endothelium.* It is this passage that allows the blood to flow rapidly through the arteries to feed the heart.

Over time you get little nicks, or little injuries, in the endothelium lining. Such an injury can be caused by high blood pressure, inhaling smoke, stress or the wrong kinds of food. In order to heal these injuries, the body has to put some kind of Band-Aid on these nicks. Actually, the Band-Aid it uses is a small cholesterol deposit.

Therefore, year after year, you have more and more of these patches of cholesterol building up in the lining of the arteries. You already know what happens eventually. The arteries fill up more and more with hardened plaque until the blood can barely pass through. I have seen autopsies of people whose arteries were so filled with this substance that cutting through their arteries was like cutting through bone.

Living Healthy Tip No. 10

"An ounce of prevention is worth a pound of cure." I believe this most strongly pertains to heart disease and cancer.

Arteriosclerosis has been called a silent killer because there are no nerve endings in your arteries, and the arteries can become clogged before we recognize any telltale signs or feel any sensation.

What's the Treatment?

More money is spent in the United States each year treating heart disease than for any other illness–a mind-boggling $78 billion a year. About $18 billion is spent on one hundred seventy thousand bypass surgeries and another $6 billion on angioplastic surgeries.

Angioplasty is a procedure using a balloon on the tip of a catheter. Your surgeon inserts it into the clogged artery and expands the balloon, breaking up the plaque so that blood can once again flow through. Bypass surgery and angioplasties, however, are not the answer to the problem of heart disease. They are simply a treatment.

We must begin to focus on the root causes of heart disease. We need to understand what causes the plaque to form in the arteries and what causes high blood cholesterol. How can we avoid foods with high fat contents and other substances that cause injury to the linings of the blood vessels?

Insurance companies pay about $30,000 for a bypass operation and about $7,500 for an angioplasty. Guess how much they pay a doctor to teach a healthy person how to prevent heart disease? Zero!

Our system is geared to treat medical problems with everything from surgery and special procedures to cholesterol-lowering drugs and medications. It seems that every week I receive an invitation from a pharmaceutical company to attend a dinner and hear about medicines that can help either heart disease or some other medical condition.

The key to having a healthy future lies not in better medications or more skilled surgeons, but in total prevention. The question you need to look into a mirror and ask yourself is this: "What can I do to reduce greatly the fat in my diet? What can I do to strengthen my heart and clear my arteries?"

In the early part of this century, heart disease was almost nonexistent in this country. Why? As individuals we did not take in the amount of fatty substances we now do.

People in undeveloped nations who cannot afford to eat steak, butter and fatty foods experience very little heart disease. Their so-called poverty diets consist of healthy fruits, grains and vegetables. Even the Japanese have one-tenth the heart problems found in this country.

The famous Coronary Artery Surgery Study in the late 1970s followed seven hundred eighty heart patients. Half of those in the sample had bypass surgeries, and the other half were treated with medicine. Here's what they found: The group that received the medicine had the exact same longevity and the same incidence of heart attack as the group that had bypass surgeries. Within five years of having a bypass, 50 percent of their arteries were clogged again. Within seven years of a bypass, 80 percent of the arteries were clogged.[1]

Obviously, for most people surgery is a temporary solution. They have a scare, but they continue eating their thick steaks and fatty foods loaded with butter and cheese.

Living Healthy Tip No. 11

When you walk in love, powerful emotions such as fear, resentment and bitterness are unable to gain a stronghold.

Some people shrug their shoulders and say, "It's hereditary. My grandpa had heart disease. My dad had it. I guess I will have it, too."

Such an attitude is walking in fear, not in faith. You need to know that in most cases heart disease is not a problem of heredity but of nutrition. It's the result of what we are taking into our bodies.

What About Cholesterol?

I am shocked when I ask people to tell me their cholesterol number. Very few know the answer. Even fewer know their *good cholesterol* and their *bad cholesterol* numbers.

You need to be aware of the fact that if your cholesterol is less than one hundred fifty, chances are slim that you will develop heart disease. The same is true if your total *cholesterol-to-HDL* ratio is less than three–it is unlikely you will have a problem. Those target numbers should be your goal.

But if your cholesterol levels are within the healthy range, it still doesn't mean you should go out and start feasting on triple-decker salami sandwiches and munching on pork rinds. Your numbers are likely to change in a hurry if you do.

In my family practice I have been asked dozens of questions about cholesterol. "Why do we have to have it?" "Is it necessary for good health?" "How can I avoid the problems connected with high cholesterol?" Cholesterol is simply a fatty, plaque-like substance that does not float around in the blood by itself. It must be connected to a protein. Actually, it is linked to two main types of protein: LDL (low-density lipoprotein) and HDL (high-density lipoprotein).

Picture a little cholesterol molecule hooked to a protein molecule that's moving around in the blood. The higher the LDL protein, the greater your chances of developing plaque in your arteries. HDL is the "good cholesterol," and the higher it is the less risk of heart disease you face.

Many researchers believe the reason LDL cholesterol is harmful is that it oxidizes and becomes toxic to cells. On the other hand, HDL cholesterol is an antioxidant and protects the blood vessels.

There is an important reason your body has cholesterol in it. It is used in the construction of the membranes of all your cells, and it forms many hormones such as testosterone, estrogen and adrenaline. Cholesterol is the raw material from which these hormones are made.

Your body produces cholesterol in the liver. People with very high cholesterol are placed on a special medicine that actually blocks its manufacture.

The average American has a cholesterol count of two hundred twenty, which is dangerously high. How large a problem is high cholesterol in the United States? Over one hundred million people–40 percent of our population (including children)–have high cholesterol. That is an epidemic by any standard.

Unfortunately, many people are placed on medicine to control this condition, yet they do not limit their consumption of harmful fats that caused the problem. If every person in the United States with high cholesterol were to take these commonly prescribed medicines, the cost would reach $300 billion a year. Again, the solution is not found in a prescription; it is found but in a changed lifestyle. I often think of the words God spoke through the prophet Hosea: "My people are destroyed for lack of knowledge" (Hos. 4:6).

Problem Foods

What foods are high in cholesterol? An egg yolk has approximately 250 milligrams of cholesterol per yolk. Also in the high category are liver, kidney, crab, lobster and shrimp. Saturated fats–those found mainly in animals–are the major culprits. Saturated fats are present in red meat, pork, animal products and in the dark meat and skin of chicken and turkey. These fats are also found in coconut oil, palm oil and in cocoa butter.

Most people consume 40 to 50 percent of their calories from fat. That is far too much. We should take in less than 30 percent of our calories from fat. Think of it! If a man takes in about three thousand calories a day (the correct caloric intake of an average man), that would be nine hundred calories of fat. When we divide that number by nine to determine the grams of fat, it equals 100 grams of fat daily.

In my opinion, we should not take in more than 30 grams per day of saturated and polyunsaturated fats. I try to target my personal intake below that number. I believe, however, that it is healthy to take in 30 percent of monounsaturated fats a day. These fats are found in olive oil, avocados, macadamia nuts, organic peanuts and almonds.

For a woman who takes in two thousand calories per day, 30 percent would be six hundred calories of fat. Divide that by nine and you would be consuming almost 70 grams per day. Women, that is far too much for your body.

Why do populations in the Mediterranean region have low incidences of heart disease? Many believe it is because they use olive oil almost exclusively. Olive oil is a monounsaturated fat that has excellent properties. I recommend that people use it on salads, in stir-fry dishes and as a substitute in any recipe that calls for oil.

Living Healthy Tip No. 12

Foods that form significant amounts of free radicals are polyunsaturated fats such as salad dressings, mayonnaise, peanut butter and other polyunsaturated fats that become rancid over time. Avoid these fats.

A Closer Look at Fat

Polyunsaturated fats

Because they are not saturated fats, many feel they can indulge freely in polyunsaturated fats or transfatty acids (found in margarine and shortenings) without a problem. That's not true at all. In most cases these can be quite harmful. Choose some of the substitute products we have mentioned throughout this volume that will not tend to clog your arteries.

Your daily diet

How much fat is in the average daily diet? The next time you are at the checkout counter of the grocery store, I suggest you pick up a fat gram counter book. You may be in for a surprise. Here are a few examples.

Item	Fat Grams
1 tablespoon of butter	11
1 tablespoon of oil	14
1 tablespoon of mayonnaise	12
1 tablespoon of salad dressing	8
1 ounce of cheddar cheese	8
1 cup of ice cream	34
1 cup of whole milk	8
T-bone steak (3 ounces)	21
Pork ribs (3 ounces)	37.5

Facts like these may be the wake-up call you need to change your eating habits. You don't have to be much of a mathematician to know that when you put five tablespoons of oil on your salad, you are taking in seventy grams–more than a two-day supply of fat.

Who eats just three ounces of ribs? A ten-ounce portion would be more common, and that would contain a total of 125 grams of fat. When you realize that ribs are 80 percent fat and 20 percent meat, you will understand they are not a healthy menu choice.

What is my daily recommended fat gram intake? No more than 30 grams a day.

Those quickie meals

Millions of people regularly eat at popular fast-food restaurants. Let's pause for a moment and see what we are really eating.

- Burger King Whopper contains 36 grams of fat. With cheese, 43 grams. Regular fries, 13 grams of fat. (The meat of a Whopper contains a lot of saturated fat.)

- McDonald's Big Mac, 32 grams of fat.
- Two slices of Pizza Hut pepperoni pizza, 23 grams of fat.
- Wendy's Big Classic with cheese, 40 grams of fat.
- Taco Bell soft chicken taco, 10 grams of fat. (Though made with chicken, it contains saturated fat.)
- One thigh of Kentucky Fried Chicken, 30 grams of fat. A small snack dinner with two pieces of fried chicken and a biscuit, 64 grams. Add a slice of apple pie, 91 grams of fat.
- Denny's Grand Slam breakfast–heralded as the most popular breakfast in the United States–with two eggs, two links of sausage, two pieces of bacon and two little pancakes, more than 1,100 calories and far too much fat.

Please don't jump to the conclusion that I am targeting McDonalds, Denny's or any other restaurant. On the contrary, each of these national chains has introduced low-fat meals and promoted them heavily. The problem lies with the customer. Americans have developed a taste for foods high in fat, and the restaurants are responding to the ordering habits of their customers.

Living Healthy Tip No. 13

The typical American diet contains excessive amounts of fat, sugar and salt and a significant lack of fiber. The key to a healthy diet is to eat primarily fruits, vegetables, whole grains, nuts, seeds, beans, legumes and lean meats.

Are you beginning to understand why we have an epidemic of heart disease?

Blood and milk?

The Masai people are cattle herders who live in Kenya in East Africa. They received a great deal of attention a few years ago when they were studied by researcher George Mann of Vanderbilt University. This tribe not only drinks whole milk from their cattle, but they also bleed the cattle and mix the milk with blood, drinking it from gourds.

Mann was intrigued because these people were eating an incredible amount of fat, yet not developing elevated levels of heart disease.

When members of the tribe died, Mann was granted permission to perform autopsies on their bodies. These tribesmen died of causes other than heart disease, but when he examined their hearts, he found their arteries to be as badly damaged as those with heart problems in the United States.

He also discovered something else. The arteries of the Masai were double the size of our arteries, because these people walked ten to twenty miles a day. Walking built up their arteries and helped them thrive, even with heart damage.[2]

Watch Those Free Radicals

Earlier we discussed the impact that free radicals have on cancer. Free radicals also play a role in heart disease. Like cholesterol, free radicals can be good. They can actually destroy bacteria, stop inflammation and help our red blood cells use oxygen.

When free radicals are in high supply, however, danger lurks. It can happen when someone is blowing cigarette smoke in your face or when your blood pressure is elevated. In such situations they bind to the LDL proteins connected to the cholesterol cells and form a foam cell. This condition leads to a fatty streak, which then leads to arteriosclerosis.

Years ago they did autopsies on the soldiers who served in Korea and found that many of the young men, about eighteen years of age, had fairly advanced arteriosclerosis. Why? Because of the stress of war, their smoking habits, their diets of foods high in fats and cholesterol and their high blood pressure. These factors created intense free radical damage because their systems were under attack.

Living Healthy Tip No. 14

Fats such as margarine, corn chips, potato chips and pastries cause free radical damage. They not only predispose you to develop heart disease but can accelerate cancer growth.

Air Pollution

When I drive past a jogger on the side of a busy road, I feel sorry for him or her. The greatest danger that person is facing is not a swerving driver, but the fact they are sucking carbon monoxide and noxious chemicals from the exhaust of cars into their lungs.

They are running for their health, yet they could be ruining it in the process. There have been times that I wanted to stop my car and warn them of their health hazard. They are unknowingly getting a whopping dose of free radical damage.

Harmful Chemicals

Pesticides, herbicides and all the other industrial chemicals we're exposed to in our diets can also cause free radicals to be formed in our bodies that can damage the linings of our blood vessels.

Silenced by Stress

"Why did I have this heart attack?" a patient wanted to know. The fifty-year-old accountant had plenty of reasons to ask.

- His cholesterol count was 137.
- His blood pressure was normal.

- He had no family history of heart failure.
- He did not smoke.
- He was not overweight.
- He exercised regularly.

Yet the man had a sudden, massive heart attack. What happened? It did not take long to determine that the coronary he suffered was the result of years of severe stress that he had experienced. How is this possible? Research shows that stress has a strong influence on the development of free radicals, and sustained stress can build to a level that causes major damage to the heart.

Prozac is one of the most commonly written prescriptions in America because so many people feel unable to cope with the stress in their lives. Looming financial demands, too little time to communicate with spouses, conflicts and crises in the workplace all contribute to feeling overwhelmed and stressed out.

Unfortunately, stress that is sustained over a long period of time soon becomes distress, which then leads to anxiety and depression. I have seen too many people who are on the edge of an emotional feeling of fight or flight. They wring their hands in fear, and when you ask what they are worried about, they respond, "I just don't know!" In a person who is depressed, all the body's systems become geared down, and he or she lives under a cloud of gloom, hopelessness and extreme sadness.

I believe we are living in the days written about in Luke, with "men's hearts failing them for fear" (Luke 21:26).

The answer to a person's depression is not found by placing our trust in man, because such misplaced trust often leads to disappointment. The joy of the Lord is our strength. We can be encouraged and lifted up by praying in the Spirit, meditating on God's Word and by praising and worshiping God. His anointing breaks the yoke of heaviness and depression.

One of the great benefits of a spiritual relationship with Jesus Christ is that you can cast your cares on the Lord and allow Him to lift your heavy burdens. Proverbs 17:22 says, "A merry heart doeth good like a medicine: but a broken spirit drieth the bones."

Lowering the Pressure

One out of four Americans has high blood pressure–that's about sixty million people. High blood pressure exerts a sheering force on the arteries, forming little injuries. Medical research has linked this condition to two factors:

1. Being overweight.
2. Taking in too much salt.

Most Americans take in 10 to 20 grams of salt a day. That's far too much. We only need about a tenth of a teaspoon of salt, yet we routinely take in two to four teaspoons a day. The recommended daily allowance for salt is about one teaspoon.

How does eating too much salt adversely affect us? Salt acts as an agent to hold water in our blood vessels. Picture a water balloon. As you fill the balloon with liquid, it increases the amount of pressure pushing against the balloon. It's the same with salt. The higher the salt content in the body, the more water that's retained and the higher the blood pressure.

Most people experience an immediate lowering of blood pressure with a decrease in salt intake. Losing weight also has a noticeable effect, because we are usually eliminating processed foods that are high in salt.

Most processed meats, such as salami and bologna, have a high salt content. Canned foods and soups need to be watched closely. One can of soup may contain over 1,000 milligrams of salt.

Fast foods are also culprits because of a simple reason: Salt makes them taste better. Salt is also found at high levels in fermented foods such as pickles and bottled sauces. One pickle can contain 1,000 milligrams of salt. Since salt acts as a preservative, you'll also find great quantities of it in butter and dairy products.

Here are additional proven ways to lower your blood pressure:

- Eat less meat and dairy products.
- Decrease your fat intake.
- Increase your calcium.
- Increase your intake of potassium (use potassium salt as a salt substitute, and eat plenty of bananas).
- Take garlic.

- Take antioxidants.
- Exercise regularly.

We cannot prevent heart disease without keeping our blood pressure low. Begin to address this problem today.

Eight Keys to Weight Loss

About 30 percent of all teenagers are from fifteen to thirty pounds overweight. I've been asked repeatedly to recommend a particular diet for weight loss. The following is more than a diet. It is a program that, if followed, will result in a lifestyle change that will not only allow you to lose weight but will help you to keep it off.

Here are the eight keys:

1. Eat breakfast like a king (a big, healthy breakfast), lunch like a prince (medium portions) and dinner like a pauper (a small meal). Do not eat past 7 P.M.
2. Avoid fried foods and limit saturated and polyunsaturated fats. Instead, choose the *good fats*–including olive oil,

avocados, macadamia nuts and organically grown peanuts. I recommend taking 1 tablespoon of flaxseed oil a day. (Keep the flaxseed oil in the refrigerator, and do not cook with it.)

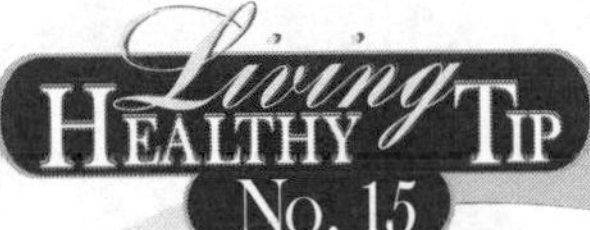

Hydrogenated fat is man-made, and it raises cholesterol levels and increases the risk of heart disease. It is found in margarine, mayonnaise, salad dressings, candy bars, potato chips, crackers and many processed foods.

3. Limit your calorie intake. Men on diets should limit their intake to between one thousand and two thousand calories a day. If you receive too few calories your body will send a signal that it is starving and will actually hold on to calories. This condition can actually cause you to gain weight.

4. Remain carbohydrate free after 3 P.M. If you want to lose weight, carbohydrates such as bread, rice, noodles, pasta and starchy vegetables are

excellent to eat. However, if you eat them late at night, they will form fat. That's why I tell my patients not to consume them after 3 P.M.

5. Exercise either four times a week for twenty minutes or three times a week for thirty minutes. The best exercise is brisk walking. Don't overexert yourself and end up huffing and puffing, because that can cause free radical damage to your body.

6. Avoid sweets, candies, chocolates or any foods containing excessive amounts of sugar.

7. Eat one banana fiber muffin every morning. (See recipe in the back of this book.)

8. Study and apply the *Carbohydrate-Protein-Fat Plan* daily. (This diet program is presented in the back of this book.)

Getting in Shape

Bodily exercise is great for you, but there are limits. For years I pushed my body very hard until I had heat stroke and almost died. It was the result of setting unrealistic goals and not allowing my body to stop when it needed to stop. Now, older and wiser, I have slowed my pace, and I listen to what my body is saying.

I have talked at length with many highly trained athletes, including marathon runners, who are compulsive exercise enthusiasts. The downside of compulsive exercise is that many of these people suffer from constant muscle soreness and chronic fatigue.

I recommend low-intensity workouts and moderation in physical exertion, because the pressure associated with excessive exercise can undo the very thing you are trying to accomplish. To maintain a healthy heart we can't sit on the couch flicking through the TV channels. It's like our automobile. If we park it in the driveway and leave the engine running, eventually problems will arise. It must be driven. In the same way, we must exercise our bodies to stay fit.

It's important to get our heartbeat up to a good training rate without going over the limit. Exercising as hard as you can is like flooring the accelerator of your car. It's not good for the engine. When you push your body too hard you are releasing tremendous amounts of free radicals into your system that can damage your heart.

You should exercise three times a week for thirty minutes or four times a week for twenty minutes. To determine your target heart rate during exercise, follow this formula. Start with the number 220 and subtract your age. Then multiply that times .65 (65%). Multiply it again times .80 (80%). The range between the two numbers is the range for which you should be aiming. Here is an example for a forty-year-old female.

TARGET HEART RATE

220 minus 40 equals 180

180 times .65 (65 percent) equals 117

180 times .8 (80 percent) equals 144

This individual should be exercising enough to reach a heart rate between 117 and 144. She should not reach 160 or 180 beats per minute because her heart could be damaged in the process.

Brisk walking is the best exercise I can recommend. You don't need expensive equipment or a membership in a health club. Simply buy a good pair of walking shoes so that you don't injure your feet, and find a soft-walking surface so you don't injure your joints.

You don't need to be huffing and puffing while you are walking or trying to keep up with someone who is walking or jogging faster. Some people find that walking the dog is the best workout they get.

Low intensity exercise helps our bodies build up their antioxidant enzyme systems. It also increases lymphatic flow, which cleanses our blood. That's why low-intensity exercise is so good for us.

Important Reminders

In an earlier chapter we discussed the importance of vitamins and minerals as they relate to cancer. They are also vital in preventing heart disease. Take plenty of vitamin E. I recommend that you should take a minimum of 400 International Units a day. Take more if you are on a regular exercise program.

Purchase natural vitamin E extracted from vegetable oil. It is called D-alpha-tocopherol. Always check with your physician. You should not add excessive amounts of vitamin E to your diet if you are taking anticoagulants or using aspirin to prevent blood clots. Why? Vitamin E can cause increased bleeding. When I perform surgery on a patient I make sure that they stop their vitamin E for at least forty-eight hours prior to surgery, because it works like an anticoagulant and keeps blood from clotting.

Vitamin C is also very important in the prevention of heart disease. We should take in at least 1,000 milligrams a day. If you are under heavy stress, or if you are participating in a heavy exercise program, double or triple that dosage.

Chewable vitamins can make your mouth so acidic that the enamel is actually eaten off your teeth. It's best to purchase vitamin C capsules that you can swallow.

For heart disease prevention, take at least

25,000 units a day of beta carotene–more when you are under stress. You may choose beta carotene instead of vitamin A.

Add 200 micrograms of the antioxidant selenium daily to protect your cell membranes from damage. Take coenzyme Q-10 to prevent free radical damage due to lack of oxygen and for angina problems. I recommend 30 milligrams twice or three times a day.

Living Healthy Tip No. 16

Jesus did not say, "If you fast," but rather "When you fast." (See Matthew 6:16.) Fasting is one of the best ways to detoxify the body and draw closer to God.

To lower your triglyceride levels, take omega-3 fats daily. They are obtained from flaxseed oil and fish oil. I recommend three fish oil gel caps three times a day with meals, or 1 tablespoon of flaxseed oil one to two times a day.

Don't forget the importance of soluble fiber. It helps prevent the absorption of cholesterol. You can get it from oat bran, rolled oats, carrots, freshly ground flax seeds and rice bran. Also consume plenty of fresh fruits and vegetables–especially beans.

Reversing the Disease

Many people tell me, "I'm too far gone. I've eaten this way for sixty years. My arteries are probably clogged, and it's too late."

That's not necessarily correct. Notable medical professions say that heart disease can be reversed, and I agree with them. Doing so will require that you become tougher on yourself. No more than 10 percent of your calories should be from fats–and no saturated fats at all. Aim for practically no cholesterol intake. That means no egg yolks, shell fish or organ meats. Cut out polyunsaturated oils and all animal products except for yogurt and skim milk. Eat a tremendous amount of fiber, both soluble and insoluble. On a more positive note, you do not have to restrict your calories. You can eat as much fruit and as many vegetables as you want. Have a complete physical every year.

The most important thing you can do to fight heart disease is ask God to help you. He desires that you have a perfect heart, both physically and spiritually.

Notes

Chapter 3

Eating to Live

RECENTLY I HEARD THE STORY OF A MAN who grew up in California. As a teenager he did a lot of fishing. Year after year he would go down to the San Francisco Bay to fish, and then he would clean and eat his catch.

One day, as he returned to his favorite fishing spot, he saw a huge sign posted. It read:

Eating fish caught in this area may be harmful to your health because of chemical contamination.

Concerned, he decided to have his blood tested. The results revealed dangerously high levels of pesticides in his body.

Pesticides, especially at elevated levels, are associated with cancer–although it's a fact that is rarely told. Consequently, unsuspecting individuals are constantly consuming foods and beverages that are laden with contaminants and pesticides that slowly but surely do them harm.

This fisherman who so enjoyed fishing in San Francisco Bay and eating his day's catch eventually ingested enough contamination to threaten his health. Without warning, he had eaten harmful substances, one bite at a time.

The Peril of Pesticides

There is a tremendous increase in pesticide pollution in our nation. Each year more than two billion pounds of harmful pesticides are spread across our land–that's about ten pounds for every man, woman and child.

Since pesticides do not break down quickly, their effects are felt for many years. In 1972, the pesticide DDT was banned. However, this substance is so difficult to eliminate that more than a quarter of a century later, traces of DDT continue to show up in many soils. It continues to be found in rooted plants such as carrots and potatoes.

What effect have pesticides had on our environment? The various kinds of pesticides we use have increased thirty-three times since 1940, and their toxicity has risen tenfold. To make matters worse, crop losses to insects and weeds have multiplied at an alarming rate, indicating that insects and weeds are becoming more resistant to modern day pesticides. Sadly, the response to these crop losses will be the additional use of even more pesticides. This year, more than two billion pounds were spread over American soil. Get ready for three, four and perhaps even ten billion pounds!

As an indication of the resistance we're encountering from pesticides, in a recent report I learned that the Environmental Protection Agency (EPA) has actually identified sixty-four pesticides to date as potentially carcinogenic or able to cause cancer.

Potentially carcinogenic means it hasn't been completely proven. It may take twenty or thirty years for the results to come in. It is my opinion, however, that we need to take personal responsibility for eliminating pesticides from our diets without delay.

Nearly everyone living in the United States–99 percent of the population–has some detectable level of pesticides in his or her body. What is the best way to reduce your intake of these harmful agents? Begin by identifying the foods that have the highest levels of these enemies, and then reduce your intake, or totally eliminate them from your diet. Let's look at some of the things that are part of our daily diets that often contain high levels of pesticides.[1]

Living Healthy Tip No. 17

Choose high chlorophyll drinks and foods such as wheat grass, barley grass, blue-green algae and chlorella. These foods help to cleanse the gastrointestinal tract and detoxify the body of heavy metals.

Water

Industrial waste and pesticides have polluted much of our water supply. Unfortunately, most people do not realize that much of our water contains potentially cancer-causing chemicals.

What water should I drink?

Many health-conscious individuals have chosen to use distilled, bottled water for personal drinking. However, it is impossible to remove all the impurities found in water by merely boiling it.

Distilled water is very inexpensive and should be used not only for drinking, but to prepare juices and for cooking. My advice is not to drink tap water. It's perfectly fine for bathing but not for drinking.

One government report identified over two thousand chemicals in our drinking water. Some water supplies when examined extensively have registered as high as sixty thousand chemicals.[2] Many water-testing facilities can only perform tests for thirty or forty chemicals. That means a test may not detect the presence of some chemicals that go beyond the range of their testing ability.

About 80 percent of Americans drink chlorinated water, yet it may not be the best alternative. When chlorine combines with organic material, it can form a chemical that is a recognized carcinogen. In addition to these chemicals in our drinking water, other industrial chemicals and radioactive materials are often present. You may wonder how fertilizer can harm our drinking water. Fertilizers contain nitrates, and when nitrates are combined with organic materials they form nitrosamines, which are also carcinogens.

Just a few decades ago, when a well was dug, pure water could be found at a depth of about fifty feet. Today in wells as deep as two hundred feet we usually do not find pure water, but water containing fertilizers and nitrates. In some areas people are digging wells as deep as four hundred feet and still finding pesticide residue. This should concern us deeply. Pure water is vital to maintaining good health.

What about water filters?

Several types of water filters are available, and I will discuss them briefly. If you drink nonchlorinated water, reverse osmosis is an excellent type of filter. It eliminates most chemical contaminants, except for certain chemicals caused from chlorine.

Distillation is also very effective, but it may not remove all the chlorine-related chemicals. Consequently, if you distill your water, make sure you use nonchlorinated water.

In my opinion, one of the best types of filtering processes is reverse osmosis with an activated charcoal filter. It removes up to 97 percent of the chlorine-related chemicals, which is considered excellent. Another fine choice is a filter with reverse osmosis and deionization.

What about bottled water?

I've been asked, "If I buy bottled water, is it pure and safe to drink?" I recently spoke with a representative of the company from which I buy my distilled bottled water. They informed me that their water is treated with reverse osmosis and activated charcoal filter and virtually all the chemicals have been removed. In other words, it is safe. But if you purchase bottled spring water, it is processed differently. In fact, bottled water is subject to the same standards as ordinary drinking water–which are often not really standards at all! That is why it is important to understand these basic principles so you can make an intelligent choice regarding the water you drink and the purification standards used.

Living HEALTHY TIP No. 18

Practice deep breathing throughout the day to oxygenate your body. You can live about seven days without water, about seven weeks without food, but only for five minutes without oxygen.

I have touched only lightly on the topic of water filters and processes. If you have a specific question about a particular water filter, you can contact The National Sanitation Foundation, East

Lansing, Michigan, or Water Quality Association, Lisle, Illinois.

Fish

Since we know that toxins and pesticides are invading our rivers, lakes and seas, we have to ask ourselves, "What is this doing to our fish?" There are a number of fish that are absorbing these pesticides and have become contaminated as a result.

With all the chemical contaminants in our lakes and rivers, no longer can we just eat from anywhere. Because pesticides are stored in the fatty tissues of the meat, when we eat fish caught in waters surrounding highly industrialized areas, we consume these stored pesticides along with the fish.

What fish should you avoid?

Avoid eating shark and swordfish. Although these two fish are expensive, they have some of the highest levels of mercury and pesticides of any fish in the sea. Sharks will eat anything, and they eat a lot of pesticides. In many areas trout have also been subjected to contamination through industrialization. Use caution, and select fish taken from fresh, pure water areas.

Keep it simple.

You can't go wrong eating orange roughy and red snapper. Although shrimp does contain higher levels of cholesterol than other seafood, it is basically free from contamination and therefore safe to eat. If you enjoy salmon, get Pacific salmon. Sole is also an excellent choice.

Tuna is another fine option because it is nearly pesticide free. You should be aware, however, that it often contains moderate levels of mercury. Albacore white tuna tend to have the lowest levels of mercury.

If you purchase your fish from a grocery store, there are certain things for which you should look. First, realize that nearly 40 percent of your grocer's fish may have already begun to spoil. You can assure the quality of your purchases by using this brief checklist.

- Fresh fish are shiny, bright and bulging.

- If it smells fishy, don't buy it.
- If the scales are shiny, the fish is good.
- If your touch leaves an indentation in the flesh, don't buy it. The flesh should spring back.
- If the fish has not been kept on ice at 32 degrees, don't buy it. It is likely that it has already begun to spoil.

In what waters are the purest fish found?

Certain waters are known for their purity. The waters of Australia are extremely pure, as are the waters of Argentina and Chile. The seas surrounding New Zealand and Iceland are also extremely clean. Nearly any type of fish you purchase from these waters should be safe to eat.

Since it is not always possible to know where your fish is from, here is a list of some fish that are almost always pesticide free:

- Orange roughy
- Red snapper
- Sole

- Pacific salmon
- Mahi-mahi (Florida)
- Trout
- Halibut
- Grouper (Argentina, Chile, Mexico)

Shellfish

The Bible, our handbook for life, contains some helpful, health-related guidelines. Leviticus 11:9–10 says: "These shall ye eat of all that are in the waters: whatsoever hath fins and scales in the waters, in the seas, and in the rivers, them shall ye eat. And all that have not fins and scales in the seas, and in the rivers, of all that move in the waters, and of any living thing which is in the waters, they shall be an abomination unto you."

Interestingly, when this scripture was written the water supply was clean. No Industrial Revolution with its factories, chemical contaminants and pesticides had yet contaminated the earth's lakes and streams. Nevertheless, this passage offers a caution about shellfish.

Some shellfish are highly polluted and should

be avoided. Until recently I assumed that all varieties of shellfish were generally considered the cockroaches of the sea and contained the highest levels of pesticides. For example, I was surprised to discover that shrimp is a varicty of shellfish that is nearly free of pesticide and industrial toxin contamination.

Other shellfish that are basically pesticide free are certain varieties of crab and scallops. If you select any of these shellfish, simply remember to eat those from less-industrialized areas where the waters remain uncontaminated.

Living Healthy Tip No. 19

The healthiest fats and oils to choose include extra-virgin olive oil, almonds, avocados, cashews, pistachios, macadamia nuts, flaxseed oil, fish oil and primrose oil.

Meats

Meats are an important part of the American

diet, but alarming questions have been raised regarding their fat content.

Animals store very large amounts of toxins, pesticides and industrial wastes in their fatty tissues. The fattier the piece of meat, the greater the potential for the storage of pesticides. Many thousands of pesticides are being sprayed on our land each year, and the cattle that graze on that land are ingesting them. These harmful substances are not only ingested by these animals, but are immediately stored in their fat. So, if you are fond of fatty pieces of meat, such as T-bone steaks or ribs, you're eating more than protein. You are transferring loads of pesticides into your body. The fattier the cut of meat, the more carcinogens it can contain.

The meat of animals, especially the fatty parts, often contains carcinogens and neurotoxins–a poisonous protein complex that acts on the nervous system–which can poison us. I believe these poisons are contributors to many of the neurological diseases common today.

Pesticides include herbicides, rat poisons, fungicides and insecticides. Many insecticides attack the nervous systems of insects and rodents. When we take in fatty meats, pesticides that may contain neurotoxins go into our own fatty tissues and can eventually work their way into our brains.

What happens? This material can actually begin to make our brains toxic by accumulating in the cells of this vital organ. We still don't understand all the problems associated with this phenomenon because we don't do studies on human brains. I believe we will eventually discover that many of these neurotoxins and pesticides are key causes of the increase of neurological diseases that we're seeing in our nation.

Think lean.

It is vital to choose lean cuts of meat. The best choice is turkey. It is not only the leanest, but it contains the least amount of pesticides and toxins. Other options include chicken, some fish and lean cuts of red meat. If you choose to eat lobster, try to select Australian or Alaskan lobster–I personally avoid eating Maine lobster because of the industrial pollution in the waters of the Northeast.

Chicken is another good choice. The cleanest chickens are called free range, which indicates they were not fed antibiotics. Free-range chickens are also raised on land that is generally not sprayed with pesticides and fertilizers. Purchasing free-range chickens from health food stores is a little more expensive. Many free-range meats and poultry are now found in grocery stores. The breast is always the best choice simply because it contains the lowest amount of animal fat.

Peel the skin off and cut away any visible fat from chicken and turkey before it is cooked. This is extremely important because if you leave the fat and skin on, the pesticides seep into the meat.

Other relatively safe meat options include the leanest cuts of lamb, pork roast, venison (U.S.), rabbit, goose, buffalo and duck. However, it is best again to choose free-range meats.

Meats that should be limited to once a week include:

- Ham
- Pork chops
- Hot dogs made from turkey and chicken (not beef or pork)

- Beef round steak
- Filet mignon

Avoid the fattier meats because they are extremely high in pesticide residue, such as:

- Veal (generally very high in pesticides if purchased at a grocery store)
- Bacon (tastes good, but it is not good for you)
- Beef and calf liver. Liver is one of the worst foods to eat. Years ago our mothers made us eat liver, thinking it was good for us because of the iron content. However, the liver filters the poisons from an animal's body, so I suggest you avoid eating it.
- Sausage (full of pesticides)
- Salami
- Bologna or sandwich meats
- Hot dogs (beef and pork)
- Fast-food hamburgers. What do we feed our children almost everyday? Fast-food hamburgers. What are we giving our children? High doses of pesticides that

increase their risk of cancer, heart disease and neurological disease.

- Ground beef (extremely high in pesticides)
- Chuck roast (also very high in pesticides)

The patio chef

Do you enjoy grilled meats with a nice char or burn on them? Let me tell you about that burn. Charred meats contain a chemical called benzopyrene–a highly carcinogenic substance. That's why I warn my patients to avoid charred meats.

But don't give away your grill. You can still enjoy the flavor of grilled meat that is prepared safely. Use charcoal instead of mesquite–a wood that contains more dangerous chemicals than charcoal. Place the charcoal on one

Living Healthy Tip No. 20

Eat meats that are leanest in fats, including turkey breast, chicken breast and lean free-range meats such as venison and elk.

side of the grill, and prepare your meat on the other side–away from the charcoal. Place the meat rack as high as possible, away from the flame. When meat cooks over charcoal, fat drips off the meat into the fire and turns into steam. The pesticides in the fat char into the meat, and so even greater amounts of carcinogen are formed.

Living Healthy Tip No. 21

Choose the leanest cuts of red meat such as extra-lean filet mignon.

You can still enjoy a steak without all the chemicals and contaminants. Talk to the owner of any health food store about purchasing meats that are free of contaminants. You can continue to eat lunchmeats also if you choose chicken or turkey varieties that contain no nitrates.

If you are still looking for a healthy alternative to meat, try tofu. Tofu–made from soybeans–is considered an excellent anticancer food. Tofu burgers are extremely good for you, and soybean hot dogs are also available.

Dairy Products

Since toxins are concentrated in the fatty tissues of animals, dairy products, which are extremely high in fat, pose a problem. The highest amounts of pesticide residues are found in butter and cheese.

Some people choose margarine instead of butter, never realizing that it contains transfatty acids associated with heart disease. I tell people to stay away from both butter and margarine because both can increase your risk of heart disease, and margarine can increase your risk of cancer. A good alternative is a commercial product such as Butter Buds.

Ice cream is very high in pesticide residue as well because it is full of fat. Whole milk, Half-and-Half and even cottage cheese are high in pesticides. High-pesticide offenders also include milk chocolate, chocolate cake and chocolate chip cookies.

Avoid whole milk and whole milk products. Instead, use skim milk and skim milk cheeses. Avoid whole milk ice cream by selecting skim milk ice cream, sherbet or low-fat frozen yogurt.

Here's a word of friendly advice: Don't allow yourself to get into bondage regarding these issues. For every food that contains fat there is a lean alternative. Just remember that the fat is where the toxins collect.

Most parents feed their children whole milk, cheese and foods coated with butter. When they are very good we reward them with chocolate. What are we really giving them? We are rewarding them with huge doses of pesticides. Combine that with hamburgers or fatty cuts of meat, and we are poisoning our children. By serving our youngsters foods that are rich in fat, we are placing them at a greater risk of developing cancer. It is critically important that you understand this information and pass it on to those you love.

Fruits and Vegetables

Although fruits and vegetables aren't nearly as potentially hazardous as meats and dairy products, they can still be tainted with pesticides. We will be addressing the issue of how to cleanse the products, because these foods are essential to your good health.

Fruits and vegetables contain vital fiber. The higher the fiber content of foods, the more toxins they bind, which are then eliminated from your system.

No–nos

The heaviest concentrations of pesticide residues are found in peanuts and raisins. That means that peanut butter and cereals with raisins may not be the best choices for our families.

Children and adults alike love peanut butter, yet many commercial brands are made from peanuts that are loaded with high levels of pesticides. However, you can go to the health food store and usually find organically grown peanuts and organically grown raisins, thereby avoiding the pesticide problem.

You can also serve your children peanut butter made from organically grown peanuts. It will taste slightly different than the commercial brands because it will be made from freshly ground peanuts that are pesticide free. But your children will soon develop a taste for it. Limit peanut butter servings to once per week, because it may contain a carcinogenic (cancer-causing) chemical called aflatoxin. Almond butter or cashew butter is a better choice.

Fruits with low pesticide levels

When considering what fruits to eat, here's the rule to remember: The thicker the peel, the safer the fruit. For example, bananas have a thick peel and have practically zero pesticides. Bananas are one of the best foods you can eat, and you don't have to purchase them from a health food store. Those offered by your neighborhood grocer are safe because of the thick peel. Oranges, tangerines, lemons, grapefruit, pineapples, watermelons and figs are also excellent. However, some fruits with a thick peel such as cantaloupes should be carefully examined because they have a very porous peel, which absorbs pesticides.

Fruits with high pesticide levels

The following fruits are high in pesticide residues because they have either a very thin peel or none at all: apples, pears, grapes, strawberries, peaches, kiwi, prunes, cherries, blackberries and blueberries. You should be careful about eating strawberries and peaches because they are often tainted with large doses of pesticides–almost one hundred different kinds of pesticide residues can be found on some of these fruits.

If you eat these fruits often, I would recommend buying the organically grown varieties. You can also purchase a special rinsing agent at a local health food store that removes pesticides from the fruit while washing the fruit with it. One may also simply wash them with Ivory Soap and rinse them well.

What are the best vegetables?

Organically grown vegetables are the best choice. But because these vegetables are usually more costly, many people feel they cannot afford them. If you use vegetables that are not organically grown, just be sure to wash them well with water and Ivory Soap. Wash your vegetables carefully and eat them together with your grains and fruit.

Someone may say, "I love salads. Can I still eat lettuce?" The answer is absolutely yes. Just peel off the first two or three layers to remove any pesticide-tainted leaves.

Some broccoli can contain higher levels of pesticides, so if you are eating a lot of broccoli you may want to purchase an organically grown variety or wash it well.

Vegetables with high pesticide levels

The two vegetables that have the highest levels of pesticides are spinach and potatoes. The outer portion of the potato is loaded with the offending substances, so make certain you wash and peel it. Your mother may have taught you that the best vitamins are found in the skin of the potato–but so are the pesticides. Because potatoes grow in the dirt, they absorb pesticides from the surrounding soil. So don't eat the potato skins unless you use organically grown potatoes.

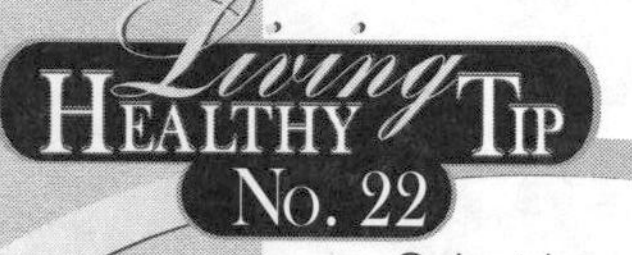

Select low-fat dairy products such as skim milk, low-fat or skim milk cheeses and yogurt.

Spinach grows near the ground, and its leaves have no protective covering, so this vegetable tends to have high concentrations of pesticides.

Moderation Is the Key

Do not get in bondage over what to eat and what not to eat. You'll do fine if you just keep it simple. Low fat is the key, and don't worry too much about your vegetables. Let your food intake be with moderation, and don't go to extremes. You do not need to stop eating at restaurants; just try to avoid fatty foods.

One obtains the most pesticides from fatty meats and only minuscule amounts from fruits and vegetables. Choose fruits and vegetables at a restaurant, and don't worry about how well they have been washed. The high fiber in the fruits and vegetables will help to bind and expel any toxins from your body.

Grains

Grains are the least toxic food in our diets. This category includes whole-grain breads, brown rice, whole-grain pastas and whole-grain cereal. The fiber in the grain traps the toxins in our colons and eliminates them.

Higher pesticide residues have been found in both white bread and whole-wheat bread. We have more than a billion pounds of pesticides spread over our farms each year, so it's sure to be on our wheat and other crops. High levels of pesticides are also found in dinner rolls and rye bread.

It is possible to find whole-wheat bread made from wheat that is organically grown. But understand that all whole-wheat bread is good for you. It will bind the toxins, and you'll excrete them. The amount of toxins that are found in these grains is small compared to the amount found in meats. Since the toxic levels found in grains are moderate, eat all you like. Fiber is good for you, and the more of it you eat the lower your chance of developing cancer because it pushes the toxins out of your gastrointestinal tract.

Beverages

Finally, I'd like to talk about the liquids you drink. Most beverages are fairly low in contaminants and pesticides if you use distilled water when preparing them. Distilled water is the key since about half the coffee we purchase has pesticides in it.

I recently learned that many of those nice white coffee filters contain dioxin, which is a very, very potent carcinogen, even in small amounts. This carcinogen is the result of the paper bleaching process. So don't buy white filters if you can find brown ones. The brown filters have no dioxin in them.

A word about soft drinks

Sodas, believe it or not, are practically pesticide free. You may, however, want to avoid Nutrasweet. While this product does not contain pesticides, chemically it breaks down to methanol, which is wood alcohol. In large doses, methanol is believed by some to be a cause of blindness. Many believe it is perfectly safe, but I do not feel drinking wood alcohol would be safe.

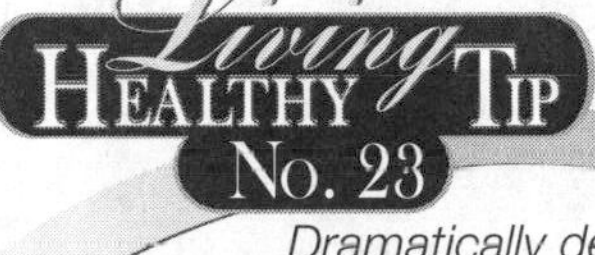

Dramatically decrease starches—including breads, crackers, bagels, pasta, rice, popcorn, corn, beans and potatoes. Excessive amounts of starches will increase insulin levels, which lead to high cholesterol, high triglycerides and eventual heart disease.

Tea is virtually free of pesticides. Make it with distilled water instead of tap water. On the other hand, wine is loaded with pesticides.

The Tragedy of Our Soil

It is unfortunate that our soil is often lacking in the vital nutrients we need to maintain our health. Since our foods do not contain all the properties necessary to sustain our bodies, we must supplement our diets with vitamins and minerals.

Why is proper nutrition vital? It helps to insure our health by giving our immune systems the ability to resist disease and sickness. When our systems become weakened through improper nutrition or environmental contamination, we become at risk for degenerative diseases and illness.

A Quick Review

The foods you want to avoid most are:

- Meats that are high in fat.
- Meats that are high in nitrites such as lunchmeats, bacon, ham, steaks, sausage and fatty cuts of meat.
- Fatty dairy products such as whole milk, ice cream, cheese and butter.
- Peanuts and raisins.

Also remember:

- When you eat fruit, choose those with a thick rind.

- When you eat vegetables, remember to include beans.
- When selecting fish, choose varieties that come from purer bodies of water.
- You can always have orange roughy and red snapper without any problems.
- Drink distilled water or reverse osmosis water.

Don't Forget Your Power Foods

The power foods listed below help to prevent disease and should be included in your diet at least once a week. It's best to eat them raw or juiced. If you prefer, you can actually steam them or make soups out of them. Be sure to drink the soup broth, because it's full of important phytonutrients, which are the cancer-fighting chemicals of tomorrow.

Eat one of the following cruciferous vegetables (vegetables in the cabbage family) at least three to six times each week: broccoli, cabbage, cauliflower, Brussels sprouts, collards, mustard greens, radishes and turnips. I suggest broccoli and cabbage as the best choices.

Carrots (or carrot juice) are also classified as power foods and are rich in beta carotene. However, if you make carrot juice, it's important to drink it as soon as possible. The longer carrot juice sits, the greater the loss of beta carotene. Drink one-half to one cup of carrot juice daily.

Tomatoes have lycopene, which is an important phytonutrient that helps in the prevention of cancer. I recommend that all men over forty-three years old eat six to ten servings a week to prevent prostate cancer.

Soybeans and soybean products are extremely powerful–perhaps one of the most important power foods. I encourage you to try soy burgers, tofu, soy protein, soy milk and miso soup. Eat one soy food every day.

Legumes, such as peas and beans, also should not be overlooked.

Parsley has very potent phytonutrients. I eat parsley a few times a week. It is a key ingredient in a Middle Eastern salad called tabouli, which is very tasty.

Chlorophyll foods–including alfalfa, wheat grass, barley grass and algae–should be taken daily. These are potent detoxifiers and have anti-tumor activity.

Strawberries are also a power food containing a very important phytonutrient.

Tangerines are a very potent power food as well, and also contain strong phytonutrients.

NOTES

WALKING IN DIVINE HEALTH
Walking in Divine Health
Walking in Divine Health
Walking in Divine Health

Chapter 4

Finding Your Way Through the Vitamin and Supplement Maze

Recently a patient walked into my office for her first visit. She weighed nearly three hundred pounds, and her chin seemed to be resting on her chest. Although only in her fifties, she had problems with arthritis, and her back was slightly bent with osteoporosis. Her walk reminded me of a cowboy in a scene from a

Western movie. I learned she could not walk quickly because of chest pains.

Upon examination I found she had angina, heart disease, high blood pressure and other obesity-related problems. The preliminary examination and tests also revealed that her cholesterol was nearly off the charts.

Trying to learn as much as possible about the cause of her health problems, I inquired, "What foods do you eat?"

"Oh, I eat the four basic food groups, and I'm sure they will keep me healthy," she responded. "I just don't understand why I gained fifty pounds over the past few years."

I asked the question again, "Tell me, what do you eat?"

She thought for a moment and settled back in her chair to tell me everything I needed to know. "Well, I fast every morning," she began. "I miss breakfast. Then for lunch I have my four food groups–a quarter-pounder with cheese, lettuce and tomato on a bun." She added, "Sometimes I have an apple pie, too. So I get my fruit."

I did not respond immediately, but considered

what this woman had just said. As you know, there are four basic food groups:

1. Meat
2. Dairy
3. Fruits and vegetables
4. Grain

She truly believed she was on target by choosing something from each group: meat–a quarter pound of hamburger; dairy–cheese; fruits and vegetables–lettuce, tomato and a slice of apple pie; and grain–a white enriched bun with sesame seeds.

It was obvious from her manner that she really thought she was eating correctly and assumed herself to be in good health.

"What do you eat for dinner?" I continued.

"Well, I'm a meat-and-potatoes woman," she told me. "I get my vegetables from potatoes, and I love T-bone steaks. So that satisfies my meat group requirement. I always include bread for my grains, and I put lots of butter on it to meet my needs for the dairy group. And I like key lime pie or lemon icebox pie for my fruit group needs."

I thought to myself, *How sad. This woman actually*

thinks she's eating healthy, when she's killing herself. I immediately surmised that the amount of fat she was consuming was setting her up for a major health crisis. Many individuals just like her have visited my office. Some have survived despite their poor habits, and some have not.

Living Healthy Tip No. 24

The average American consumes one hundred seventy pounds of refined sugar per year. About 75 percent of the sugar is hidden, and 20 percent of our diets are composed of white sugar or sucrose. This is extremely dangerous since sugar actually feeds cancer.

The survivors are those who have changed their eating habits. It is not possible to eat as this woman does and stay healthy.

Strength, Not Weakness

Most people think growing old is a natural process, yet for many the aging process is simply symptomatic of a vitamin and mineral deficiency.

The Bible says that Methuselah lived to be 969

years old. How could a man live so long? Why is it that the Bible patriarchs of old had such longevity? Scripture states that when Moses was one hundred twenty years old he was strong, energetic, and his eyesight was excellent (Deut. 34:7). Joshua and Caleb were in their eighties when they entered the Promised Land. They were still fighting battles and leading their troops–they were not so debilitated and weak that they could barely make it to their destination. They walked in with strength and vigor.

All these men of God were strong in old age, not weak. How did they do it? They obeyed God's laws and therefore lived in divine health.

Years ago, Dr. Weston Price, a dentist, visited primitive cultures throughout the world. He studied the people and their diets. He noted that when these cultures changed from their traditional diet of plants, vegetables and fruits to what was considered a more civilized diet, great changes occurred.[1]

This dentist followed the health of his subjects for approximately twenty to thirty years–especially regarding their mouths and teeth. He was able to document the onset and progression of degenerative disease in these societies that had not existed before these dietary changes.

Two other doctors became involved with Dr. Price's study. Dr. Burkett continued his research, and Dr. Trowell observed four stages through which the people progressed as they moved from the culture's traditional diet to Western eating habits.[2]

During the first stage when minimal foreign foods were introduced, there were a few cases of degenerative diseases that occurred, including mild forms of arthritis, heart disease, diabetes and cancer. During the second stage, which included more of our foods, cases of obesity and diabetes became more frequent.

During stage three they began noting many more cases of constipation, varicose veins, appendicitis and hemorrhoids due to the decreased fiber in their diet.

As these people changed to a totally Western diet, the doctors witnessed the entire spectrum of degenerative diseases common in Western society including arthritis, diabetes, obesity, cancer and heart disease.

We know what is causing our health problems.

It is the kinds of foods we eat and the environment in which we live. But what are our solutions?

I believe we can prevent many common degenerative diseases by following some basic principles outlined in this book. Why do I believe this is so? Most of these problems can be linked to marginal or moderate vitamin and mineral deficiencies, as well as eating the forbidden foods: fats, sugars and salts.

The Problem of Food Storage

Often the danger in food is not the food itself, but how it has been stored or preserved. Many people do not realize that the vitamin content of stored foods can decrease more than 70 percent over prolonged periods. For example, stored grapes can lose 30 percent of their B vitamins; stored tangerines can lose up to half of their vitamin C. Asparagus stored for one week can lose 90 percent of its vitamin C.

Much vitamin loss in fresh produce can be avoided by storing refrigerated foods at forty degrees. Frozen foods should be kept below zero degrees to retain maximum vitamin content. Unfortunately, freezing meats can also destroy up to 50 percent of thiamin and riboflavin and 70 percent of pantothenic acids.

Never store leftover meats in the refrigerator longer than three days, since this a primary cause of food poisoning. Often people who think they have the flu are actually suffering from food poisoning from eating improperly stored leftovers.

People purchase fresh fruits and vegetables, and then store them for days and weeks, not realizing that in the process much of the vitamin and mineral content is being lost.

What about processed foods? Food processing is another major cause of nutrient loss. Let me give you a few examples. Blanching, a common method of processing fish and vegetables, destroys up to half of the thiamin, riboflavin, niacin and vitamins C and B_6. Grain processing often involves removing the germ in the outer layers, and subsequently losing more than 80 percent of the magnesium. Milling cereal results in the loss of over half of its B_6 vitamin. Pasteurizing milk causes large losses of vitamin C and the B vitamins.

The more a food is processed, the higher its fat, sugar and salt content is likely to be. In addition, processing strips away valuable vitamins, minerals and fiber. We're receiving the worst and losing the best by processing our foods.

Cooking foods also causes the nutrients to be lost. What happens when you boil vegetables? As they cook, vitamins are leached out of the vegetables into water. By the time the vegetables are tender enough to eat, the mineral and vitamin content of the water is greater than that of the vegetables. Cooking causes the loss of vitamin C, B_1, B_2, niacin, B_6, selenium, potassium, magnesium, phosphorus and pantothenic acid.

Living Healthy Tip No. 25

Eating too much sugar is related to degenerative diseases—including obesity, diabetes, heart disease and arthritis.

What's the solution? Cook food in a minimal of water for a very short period of time. Also avoid chopping up your fruits and vegetables–which also contributes to the loss of vitamins and minerals.

When you cut up fruits and vegetables, you expose them to air, and they begin to lose vitamin C, folic acid, B_{12}, biotin and vitamins D, E, K and A. If you must chop or cut up your vegetables, do so just before eating them when the nutritional value will be at its optimum.

Are You Nutrient Poor?

We need approximately fifty or more nutrients to maintain our good health. Because some physicians recommend high quantities while others suggest lower amounts, I suggest that you consult your personal physician regarding what specific nutrients you may need to maintain your health and well-being.

Fifty nutrients are needed for the optimum functioning of our bodies. These include thirteen essential vitamins, twenty-two essential minerals, eight amino acids, two essential fatty acids and five cofactors. All of these nutrients interact in the body to maintain good health.

Since our cells are being renewed constantly, their quality will be determined by our nutrient intake. Nutrients also help cells to provide energy, resist disease and support the immune system.

Therefore, if you are taking in poor-quality nutrients, such as those found in white bread, red meat, fat-laden cheese, butter and other similar foods lacking the proper vitamins and minerals, these vitamins will become a part of your body. This will ultimately affect your health and impact your resistance to disease.

The next time you're about to cut into a piece of chocolate cake or take a bite of your favorite fast-food chain's fried chicken, ask yourself, "Do I really want that to become a part of my body?"

Every day cancer cells, or abnormalities, have the potential to form within us. Fortunately our incredible immune systems have a surveillance strategy to identify these cells. Once they are identified, a special targeting system begins to pump out killer T-cells. T-cells destroy cancer cells, and then phagocytes–other white blood cells–come later and clean up the mess. That's how our immune systems function.

We are constantly exposed to air pollution, cigarette smoke, stress and toxins in our food and water supply, so we're forming free radicals every day. If we have the proper nutritional intake, our immune systems can identify these cancer cells and totally eliminate them. However, if we are eating foods that adversely affect our immune systems by preventing them from functioning at optimum ability, then our immune systems may not be able to identify and eliminate cancerous cells.

The Modified Food Guide Pyramid

Instead of attempting to maintain good health by eating from the four basic food groups, as did the overweight woman we mentioned earlier in this chapter, there's a better way to think about consuming the right foods. It's called The Food Guide Pyramid. I have modified the Food Guide Pyramid by placing fruits and vegetables at the base instead of grains, cereals and breads.

Picture a pyramid that is made up of the recommended foods we should eat. At the base of this pyramid will be the largest amount of what we should consume. Then, as the pyramid gets higher, it narrows–symbolizing that we should eat less and less of these foods. Let's take a closer look at this food guide and how to apply it to our daily diets.

Living Healthy Tip No. 26

Eat more fresh fruit, steamed, stir-fried or raw vegetables, salads with extra-virgin olive oil and vinegar, lean meats and nuts including almonds, unsalted cashews and organic peanuts.

At the base of the pyramid are fruits and vegetables. These items should form the largest part of your diet. At least 35 percent of our food intake should be from fruits and vegetables. It is sad but true that most children eat very few vegetables on a daily basis. If your children refuse to eat them, make certain they are at least receiving a multivitamin and multimineral supplement along with chewable fruit and vegetable tablets. We should all have three to four servings of vegetables a day and two to four servings of fruit daily.

The second tier of our pyramid is made up of grains, cereals and breads. These items should comprise 20 to 30 percent of your total diet. You should consume your grains before 3 P.M. if you are trying to lose weight. Select whole grains instead of white flour or processed foods. Have two to three servings of whole grains a day in order to get their fiber. Having two banana fiber muffins a day, at midmorning and midafternoon, will provide two servings of grain. (See the recipe for banana fiber muffins in the back of the book.)

At the third tier on our way up the pyramid are meat and dairy products. The triangle is getting smaller, so the percentages are less. Meats should be approximately 10 percent of your diet, and the same for products from the dairy. I recommend that you choose fish, chicken breast and turkey breast. Limit your intake of red meat and pork.

Again, the dairy products you consume should include skim milk, low-fat yogurt, and low-fat cheeses–about two to three servings per day. Limit your meat to about four to six ounces of very lean meat or the fish previously recommended.

At the top of the pyramid are fats, oils and sweets. They are in the smallest part of the structure because they are the most dangerous substances.

We need to limit our intake from this category to less than 5 percent of our total diet. Most Americans take in over 40 percent of their calories as fats and oils, when their intake should be less than 5 percent.

What Is in Your Vitamins?

"Give me a vitamin; I want some energy!" is what people are heard to say. Vitamins are not pep pills, they're not caffeine, and they are not going to give you instant energy. Yes, they do function in the body with carbohydrates, proteins and fats to supply energy, but they are not energy pills. Instead they are part of a vital process. Vitamins are actually components of an enzyme system that functions to create energy.

The vitamin and multivitamin business is a multibillion-dollar industry, and it is possibly one of the most confusing ones we will ever encounter. Listed on a vitamin bottle are words like *milligrams* and *micrograms* that can be intimidating. With time, however, your storehouse of knowledge will increase, and such words will find a place in your daily conversations.

We need only a small amount of most vitamins to maintain good health. For instance, we require only two millionths of a gram of B_{12} a day, and the blood contains five billionths of a gram per liter. So all we need is a tiny speck of B_{12}. But what happens if we don't get that speck over weeks and months? If we lack just that tiny amount, the myelin sheaths–which form the protective covering over nerves–will deteriorate and lead to the destruction of the nerves. Our red blood cells will not have the materials they need as well–the basic components for manufacturing the blood cells. Not having that tiny speck of B_{12} will interfere with DNA synthesis. The blood cells will become larger, and even appear larger, and yet they will be fewer in number. A lack of B_{12} will also cause anemia. If we don't have that tiny speck of B_{12}, it can eventually lead to death.

An iron deficiency acts in much the same way. The body will continue to produce the red blood cells, but iron is essential in their formation. If the body is iron poor, it will manufacture little tiny red blood cells in decreased numbers.

Our bodies are so amazing that even if they

don't have enough iron or don't have enough B_{12}, they will continue to produce the red blood cells. But these cells will be defective, less in number, more easily destroyed, more easily affected by free radicals and more easily damaged. That's why it's critical that our vitamin and mineral needs are satisfied every day through our foods and through food supplements.

There are thirteen vitamins, but they simply cannot be manufactured by our bodies in the amounts necessary to sustain life. We must get them from our foods or from multivitamin supplements. How are we to get these essential vitamins when we destroy them by the way we store our food, by the way we cook our food and by the way we process our food? How can we be certain we are getting the proper vitamins?

First let's examine the two basic types of vitamins. There are fat-soluble vitamins: vitamins A, D, E and K; and there are water-soluble vitamins: vitamin C and the eight B vitamins, which are B_1, B_2, niacin, B_6, folic acid, B_{12}, pantothenic acid and biotin.

Perhaps you are under the impression that if

you are faithfully taking an over-the-counter multiple vitamin you are satisfying your daily requirements. You are not. You're not getting all the necessary vitamins. Some of the most popular varieties do not include vitamin K, and others contain the necessary vitamins but not in the proper amounts or proportions.

Opinions will always differ on what vitamins and minerals to take and on the amounts necessary. Before making any dramatic changes in the amount of vitamins or minerals you add to your daily diet, always consult your personal physician. Let your doctor determine how this modification will affect your overall health based on your individual medical history.

Living Healthy Tip No. 27

Take a fiber supplement such as freshly ground flaxseeds—five teaspoons of flaxseeds ground in a coffee grinder with eight ounces of water, taken in the morning and possibly again at bedtime. This contains the fiber and the essential fatty acids needed on a daily basis for health.

What dosage?

Vitamins have different functions. Antioxidants, vitamin A or beta carotene, vitamin E and vitamin C are the ones we're hearing the most about right now. In my opinion we should take in about 25,000 units of beta carotene once or twice a day.

I also recommend that you take 400 units a day of natural vitamin E to replace what has been lost in the processing of the grains we eat. I'm also a believer in taking at least 1,000 milligrams a day, or even more, of vitamin C. There is nothing wrong in taking beta carotene, vitamin C and vitamin E in separate tablets in addition to your daily multivitamin. You can also purchase an antioxidant vitamin that contains all three.

Regarding the family of B vitamins, the one found least often in multivitamin tablets is biotin, although it is easily available in health food stores. It's best to take the B vitamins in a water-soluble form throughout the day. If you take an over-the-counter multiple vitamin tablet, you probably take it once a day. It's better to distribute your intake of

B vitamins to a variety of intervals throughout your day.

If you are not receiving enough folic acid from a good supply of dark green, leafy vegetables, romaine lettuce, orange juice and broccoli, be sure you take it as a supplement. Folic acid is especially important for children and pregnant women. It is necessary for the repair of DNA, which decreases birth defects.

Most individuals get plenty of vitamin D in their milk. Look for the statement *vitamin D fortified* on the skim milk you purchase. You also get vitamin D from sunlight, but as we get older, our bodies become less able to convert sunlight into this essential vitamin, so we must rely on food supplements. Most multivitamins contain plenty of vitamin D.

Living HEALTHY TIP No. 28

Perform aerobic exercise such as brisk walking, cycling and swimming for a least twenty or thirty minutes three to four times a week.

Other needed nutrients

Vitamin-like substances called *cofactors* are very similar to vitamins, but the body can actually manufacture them. However, if our bodies don't have enough of the raw materials and nutrients to make them, we're going to be deficient. An extremely effective one is choline–found in egg yolks, wheat germ and liver. Not many people eat egg yolks because doctors have been warning us about their high cholesterol content. We also don't eat wheat germ because it's been removed from the bread we buy. In addition, I do not recommend eating organ meats.

If you have enough B_{12}, folic acid and methionine, your body can actually make the choline you need. If you do not have these in sufficient quantities, you are going to need about 500 milligrams of choline a day. Be sure choline is in your multivitamin.

We have mentioned the need for coenzyme Q-10–found in salmon, mackerel and sardines. Because many people do not like fish, they do not get enough of this important element. Coenzyme

Q-10 is a vital antioxidant that is very good for the heart. It also helps to synthesize some of the blood cells' proteins. You can safely take about 30 milligrams a day.

The Mineral Mine

In the Book of Genesis, Adam and Eve's diet consisted of vegetables and fruits, and they could have lived forever. But when they sinned, the ground became cursed, and it began to die. If you analyze our soil today, you will discover from the lack of nutrients that the process of death is nearly complete.

When we discussed how–beginning in the 1940s–phosphorus, nitrogen and potassium became the fertilizers added to our soil, we did not mention that although the crops were lush and beautiful, the remaining minerals kept leaching out of the ground until there were virtually none left. Literally, we've been sucking the soil dry. Today many soils are practically depleted of selenium, chromium, molybdenum and many other vital minerals.

What is the result? Because of our mineral deficiencies, we are suffering from diseases that should be decreasing instead of increasing: osteoporosis, arthritis, heart disease and cancer. We now consider these diseases to be a part of the normal aging process, but it should not be so.

What do minerals do?

Minerals form bones, and they assist in energy production, muscle contraction, blood formation, conduction of electrical impulses, building proteins, transporting substances in and out of cells and regulating the pH of the body. There are twenty two essential minerals we must have daily (possibly more). Unfortunately, most of our bodies are deficient in at least some of these.

The seven macro-minerals (which are the major minerals) are calcium, phosphorus, sodium, chloride, magnesium, potassium and sulfur. We generally get plenty of phosphorus, sodium, chloride, potassium and sulfur but not enough calcium and magnesium.

There are fifteen trace minerals: boron,

chromium, cobalt, copper, fluoride, iodine, iron, manganese, molybdenum, nickel, selenium, silicon, tin, vanadium and zinc. We obtain some of these through normal sources. For example, you don't have to rush out and get a fluoride supplement. You get it in your toothpaste and tap water. We also get also iodine from iodized salt and from fish.

We do not need a supplement for nickel, tin or vanadium. However, we need to look more closely at some others because so many people are lacking in them.

The major minerals are calcium and magnesium, and other trace minerals exist as well. Our bodies contain potentially toxic minerals such as lead, arsenic, aluminum and mercury. Some people include these in their mineral preparations, but I would not recommend you take aluminum since it is associated with Alzheimer's disease. And, of course, I do not recommend that you take mercury, lead, arsenic, cesium or radioactive minerals.

It is commonly known that as early as 3000 B.C. people in China with enlarged necks–a condition called goiters–were treated with seaweed. They would eat it for the iodine it contained, and it is said that it helped alleviate the condition.

Today, because our soil is depleted, we are lacking in many minerals our ancestors took for granted, and we are attempting to obtain them in a variety of ways. High-fiber foods can act to decrease our absorption of minerals. Some people eat a high-fiber muffin and then take a supplement pill with calcium, magnesium, iron and zinc and say, "I just had a fiber muffin, and I had my minerals. I'm fine."

However, high-fiber foods may have caused the minerals you've ingested to become bound or unable to be digested and distributed throughout your body. Instead of being absorbed, they will be excreted. Therefore it's important when you take your minerals that you do not take them with a

Living Healthy Tip No. 29

Drink two to three quarts of filtered or distilled water a day.

high-fiber supplement, or you can defeat the entire purpose.

Bless your bones!

Of the seven major minerals, the ones we lack most are calcium and magnesium. We have an absolute disease epidemic in the United States due to the lack of calcium–it is called osteoporosis. Women are affected the most. One out of every two females and one out of every four males over the age of fifty have osteoporosis–it is often called *brittle bone disease.*

I cannot count the number of times representatives from various pharmaceutical companies have come to my office to inform me about drugs that help form new bones. It is my conclusion, however, that we don't need new drugs–we simply need good diets.

Why should you pay $100 a month the rest of your life for drugs that will aid in bone formation when you can achieve the same results with proper nutrients that will also make you feel better, give you energy and protect your immune system?

One of the major causes of osteoporosis is the lack of calcium in our diets. The recommended daily allowance for calcium in children from ages one to ten is 800 milligrams a day. How much is that? A cup of skim milk has about 300 milligrams, so if your child has one cup of skim milk, he's not getting enough calcium. Children and young adults, ages eleven to twenty-four years, need 1,200 milligrams a day. If your child is in the growth-spurt age of twelve, thirteen or fourteen years old, without giving him or her 1,200 milligrams of calcium a day (about four cups of milk), his or her growth could likely be stunted. The same amount is contained in three cups of yogurt or six ounces of skim milk cheese.

How much do you need?

You can assimilate calcium in a number of ways, including taking antacid tablets made for indigestion, such as Tums. Each tablet contains

200 milligrams of calcium. The label says 500 milligrams of calcium carbonate, but of that you only get 200 milligrams of pure calcium.

From age twenty-five to menopause you need 800 milligrams of calcium daily. That's quite a bit, and I can assure you that very few women are getting that much calcium. As a result their skeletons are shrinking. My own grandmother lost six inches in height, and I have seen patients who have lost a full foot of height by the vertebra compressing due to calcium loss.

Women in their seventies and eighties walk into my office with their backs bent over and with their rib cages actually sitting on their hip bones. The problem can be corrected, but not if an individual waits until it's so far advanced that there is little bone left.

The first bones to be affected by osteoporosis are the jawbone and the vertebra in the back. That's why we have so much periodontal disease after fifty. These bones literally begin to be absorbed back into the body, and people start losing their teeth–due to a lack of calcium.

Additional sources of calcium include tofu,

greens, spinach, broccoli and navy beans. However, let me give you a word of caution regarding spinach. It does contain calcium, but it also has oxalate in it that binds the calcium and causes it to be excreted into the bowels. Therefore, don't expect to get all the calcium you need from spinach.

In addition to calcium, there are other minerals that are very important in the formation of bone. They include zinc, magnesium, copper, manganese, fluoride, silicon, boron and vitamin D.

If you think that taking an antacid table (such as Tums) is sufficient for the proper formation of bone, remember that you need vitamin D (400 international units a day), plus all the minerals previously mentioned. This is the reason that I recommend giving children a good multivitamin, multimineral, a calcium supplement and a handful of nuts to supply magnesium every day.

Many calcium supplements are available over the counter including calcium carbonate, calcium phosphate, calcium lactate and calcium gluconate. If you are on a restricted budget, however, use Tums.

Calcium citrate is more easily absorbed by the body than calcium carbonate, but it does not deliver as much of the minerals you need. Many vitamins contain calcium citrate, and I have heard people say that taking dolomite and bone meal is how they get their calcium. You may get your calcium, but you will also be getting lead, so it's best to avoid bone meal and dolomite.

Living Healthy Tip No. 30

Sleep at least seven to eight hours a night.

Chelated calcium is a good form, and it is easily absorbed. When treating people for osteoporosis in my office, I use microcrystalline hydroxyapatite concentrate (also called MCHC). It's mouthful, but MCHC is an extract of whole, raw, young animal bone. It contains not only calcium, but it also has phosphorus, magnesium, fluoride, zinc, copper and manganese. That is a good complex of minerals to help form bone.

The Problem of Acids

I believe it is best to combine calcium with vitamin D, copper, magnesium, manganese, fluoride, silicon and boron. Often a person may get enough calcium, but continue to suffer with osteoporosis because they're not receiving these other trace minerals.

We also lose calcium because of the acidic foods that we eat. For example, if you eat a lot of protein such as is found in cheese and other dairy products, your body can become acidic and your pH will start to drop. Your body will take calcium from your bones to raise the pH so that this imbalance is stabilized. Eating acidic foods actually causes calcium to be leeched from the bones to raise the pH. Older bodybuilders have a problem because of this, as do individuals who exercise a great deal. Protein foods are also acidic foods–fried foods, cheese, butter, oil, sugar and ice cream. These foods make the body acidic, which causes calcium to be pulled out of the bones to buffer the acid and raise the pH level of the body.

Neutral foods include rice, lettuce, turkey, fish,

eggs, oatmeal, apples and bananas.

Alkaline foods, which are basic foods, include grapefruit, limes, tangerines, watermelon, cantaloupe, honeydew, broccoli, garlic, sweet potatoes and lentils. You might not consider grapefruit to be alkaline, but they are. Alkaline foods actually raise the pH and prevent calcium from being leeched out of the bones, together with the other alkaline foods we have mentioned.

Diets that are high in fats and sugar also create an acidic environment that will take the calcium out of your bones. Avoid acidic foods whenever possible. Too much salt can also cause the body to lose calcium.

Soft drinks and caffeine have the same effect. Drinking them tends to raise the amount of phosphorus in the body because they are often loaded with this mineral. The body works to reestablish the one-to-one balance between calcium and phosphorus. So when the phosphorus is raised in the body and in the blood, the body will pull calcium out of the bones to raise the calcium level and achieve the balance. Consequently, when you drink soft drinks or eat a lot of phosphorus-rich foods, you are actually causing calcium to be taken out of your bones.

The typical American diet has a calcium-to-phosphorus ratio of one to two, or even one to four–because of all the high phosphorus foods and carbonated drinks we take into our bodies. We're eating up our bones by taking calcium out.

What About Antacids?

Many antacids cause loss of calcium because of the effects of the aluminum they contain. Tums, mentioned earlier, contains no aluminum and helps to add calcium.

We often have upset stomachs because we don't take in enough enzymes in our foods. Remember that if you do not eat uncooked, fresh fruits and fresh vegetables, you are not realizing the benefits from the enzymes they contain. If you cook your fruits or vegetables, you destroy their enzymes, and you must depend fully upon your own pancreatic enzymes for digestion. As a result, you experience more bloating, indigestion, heartburn and belching. This is one of the reasons

Americans are dependent upon antacids.

Why is the aluminum found in some antacids a problem? It depletes phosphorus, which then causes calcium to dissipate. To keep our bones strong we need not only to have the calcium, but also the other nutrients mentioned earlier.

Living Healthy Tip No. 31

The best way to prevent anxiety and depression—the two most common psychological disorders—is to walk in love. Read 1 Corinthians 13 two to three times a day.

Another Approach

Our bones can also be strengthened through exercise. We need to do calisthenics, brisk walking, slow jogging or weight lifting to put positive pressure on our skeletons and help to maintain the calcium in our bones. If you become a couch potato, your muscles and bones will slowly melt away.

We have three pounds of calcium in our body, and 99 percent of it is found in our bones. Only 1 percent is found in our blood streams. When this 1 percent of calcium is not supplied in our diets on a daily basis, the blood will steal it from our bones. It's the rob-from-Peter-to-pay-Paul syndrome. To avoid calcium deficiency and loss, you must take calcium daily. You can't say, "This is my one day a month or my one day a week to take calcium." It must be faithfully ingested every day.

The best time to take calcium and other minerals is at bedtime. They are absorbed into the body much better during the periods of rest.

Magnesium is the another major mineral we must have for good health. Its function is very similar to that of calcium in the process of bone formation. Magnesium also aids in the relaxation of muscles and helps in the conversion to energy of carbohydrates, proteins and fats. It helps manufacture protein and assists in creating our genetic material. Marginal deficiencies of this mineral are quite common.

Natural sources of magnesium include nuts, beans, peas, whole-grain breads, cereal, soybeans and dark green, leafy vegetables. When you look at this list, it's easy to see why many of our generation's children do not have enough magnesium in their bodies.

Two tablespoons of peanut butter have 60 milligrams of magnesium, and the same amount is found in one banana. We need about 400 milligrams of magnesium each day. Remember to buy peanut butter made from organically grown nuts. Regular peanut butter is full of pesticides.

One cup of milk has about 40 milligrams of magnesium. It's difficult to get the required amount of magnesium solely from our foods, so we need to depend on supplements.

Tiny but Mighty Minerals

Trace minerals, containing only minute amounts of minerals, are required in the diet to maintain health. They are vital to numerous chemical processes in the body. Let's talk about a few of them.

Boron

Boron is essential for normal calcium and bone

metabolism. It's found in fresh fruits, fresh vegetables and in nuts. Most people–especially children–do not get the amount necessary for their well-being. We need about 3 milligrams of boron a day. Without it we will experience changes similar to those occurring with osteoporosis.

I have found very few vitamin supplements or vitamin-mineral supplements that contain boron. When you choose a supplement, be sure it is there.

Chromium

To help maintain normal blood-sugar levels, regulate insulin and reduce deficiencies linked with diabetes, take chromium. Sources include whole-grain breads and cereals. We should take about 200 micrograms per day. This is another element that is inadequate in most multivitamin and mineral supplements.

Cobalt

We have plenty of cobalt in our system as long

as we take a multivitamin with B_{12}—which is cobalamin.

Copper

Copper is another trace mineral to search for on the label of your multivitamin and multimineral tablets. You can also get it from whole-grain bread, cereals, nuts, beans, peas and dark green, leafy vegetables.

Copper deficiency is related to a decrease in energy production, a decline in immune function and diminished concentration. I am convinced that many children who have been diagnosed with attention deficit disorder simply have trace mineral deficiencies. It's likely that many of these youngsters suffer from marginal deficiencies of copper. If your children aren't eating the foods we have mentioned, choose a supplement that contains this mineral.

Iron

The presence of iron is very important in the

red blood cells and in the prevention of anemia. Individuals with iron-deficiency anemia suffer from severe fatigue. High levels of iron in men are associated with heart attacks. Therefore, men do not need to take iron supplements. If you do, take very small amounts.

Many women are deficient in iron, but most multivitamins contain an adequate supply. Iron is also found in red meat, molasses, beans, peas and dark green vegetables.

Manganese

Don't confuse manganese with magnesium. They are different. Deficiencies of manganese are associated with weakness, growth retardation and bone malformations. We usually have an adequate supply of manganese in multivitamins and mineral supplements. You can find this trace mineral in spinach, tea, beans, peas, nuts, whole-grain breads and cereals.

Molybdenum

Most of our multivitamin and mineral preparations do not provide an adequate amount of molybdenum. Its best sources are vegetables, fruits and grains, but since it is dependent largely upon the soil, much of this mineral has been lost because of soil depletion. We need about 45 to 150 micrograms per day of molybdenum.

Nickel

We generally have adequate levels of nickel and should not seek more. Too much nickel is associated with cancer and heart disease.

Selenium

Selenium helps to protect cell membranes from free radical damage and enhances our immune systems. It is a very important mineral because it actually constitutes part of the glutathione peroxidase antioxidant system, which is one of the most potent enzyme antioxidant systems in the body.

Selenium deficiency is associated with an increased risk of cancer and increased risk of cardiomyopathy–a disease of the heart muscle causing weakness of the heart. We find this mineral in whole wheat, brown rice and oatmeal, but only if these products are grown in soils containing adequate amounts of selenium. From whatever source, we need about 100 to 200 micrograms a day.

Living HEALTHY TIP No. 32

Emotions such as fear, anger, bitterness, guilt, resentment, hatred and shame slowly weaken our bodies and our immune systems. We must love and practice forgiveness.

Silicon

The second most abundant element in nature behind oxygen is silicon. The earth is filled with it. But still there are people who are deficient in it. Why? Because silicon is lost when food is processed.

Sources of silicon include whole grains and organ meats (which I do not recommend that you eat because they're so filled with cholesterol and pesticides). Algae is a wonderful source of silicon and most other trace minerals. In fact blue-green algae contains most of the minerals one needs.

Tin

We get enough tin from the residue that reaches us from tin cans. No additional supplement of this mineral is necessary.

Vanadium

Vanadium is essential for growth in animals, but the amounts have not been established for human beings.

Zinc

A deficiency of zinc is associated with skin problems, dermatitis and healing problems. Sources of zinc are lean meats, poultry and fish. We usually find adequate zinc in our multivitamin or mineral tablet.

Other trace minerals in our body are aluminum, arsenic, cadmium, lead and mercury.

Again, we do not want to take these as a mineral supplement because they are poisonous to us.

Choosing a Multisupplement

Most multivitamins contain only twelve vitamins, and many of them lack vitamin K. When you purchase a vitamin supplement, be sure that it contains vitamin K. You may want to choose a multivitamin you can take two to three times a day. In that way you can get your B vitamins throughout the day instead of one larger dose. B vitamins are water-soluble and are best taken at intervals.

If you're an individual who tends to be allergy prone, you may want to get a hypoallergenic vitamin that doesn't have food coloring or preservatives in it. They also contain hypoallergenic fillers.

Choosing a mineral supplement is a little more difficult than choosing a vitamin supplement, and sometimes more costly. Yes, you can spend five dollars and save some money, but are you truly receiving what you need? Personally, I would choose a better mineral that is chelated rather than one that contains mineral salts.

We spoke earlier about chelation, but regarding minerals it is a process of wrapping a mineral with an organic molecule such as an amino acid that increases the absorption dramatically. Chelated vitamins and minerals are fairly new. Most vitamins still have mineral salts and do not have as good absorption qualities. The chelated versions are primarily sold in health food stores.

A word of caution regarding colloidal minerals: Many of these have extremely high amounts of aluminum in them. They may also contain mercury, arsenic and other toxic minerals.

In addition, try to choose a properly balanced nutrient ratio. The ratio of copper to zinc, for example, should be about one to ten to prevent copper malabsorption. Many minerals are not present in adequate amounts. This is especially true of calcium and magnesium supplements. We need 400 milligrams of magnesium each day.

Regarding calcium, premenopausal women need about 1,000 milligrams of calcium a day, and postmenopausal women need about 1,500 milligrams of calcium per day. Men need about 800 milligrams per day.

When choosing a multimineral supplement, examine the label carefully to be sure it has enough calcium, magnesium, boron, molybdenum, selenium, silicon and chromium.

To get one multivitamin or multimineral that contains absolutely everything you need could make it as big as a golf ball. A better option is taking additional supplements of the particular elements you truly need.

As an affordable approach, start with an over-the counter multivitamin. You may also want to supplement with biotin, or eat foods that are high in this substance. These include oatmeal, soybean, cereals and bananas. Take a complete multimineral supplement as well. And don't forget Tums, because they're very inexpensive. Take beta carotene (about 25,000 units a day), vitamin C (approximately 1,000 milligrams a day) and vitamin E (about 400 units a day).

Your total cost for all of these minerals should be about ten to fifteen dollars a month, and you'll have the basic raw materials to prevent disease without experiencing a significant financial impact upon your budget.

Test your vitamins to determine if the capsule breaks down adequately. Drop it in a glass of water. Recently I saw a demonstration that was amazing. One multivitamin I was taking took a surprising forty-five minutes to break down totally. You can also do the same test with vinegar. One woman told me she had placed one of her vitamins in vinegar and waited for hours. It still had not dissolved. She immediately switched to another brand that dissolved in only a few minutes. Don't spend your money for vitamins that don't dissolve. It can literally be money down the drain.

Living Healthy Tip No. 33

In order to lose weight, eat breakfast like a king, lunch like a prince and dinner like a pauper.

To Sum It Up

- Eat the power foods as often as possible–preferably daily.
- Concentrate on a low-fat diet, preferably less than 30 grams of fat per day and less then 10 grams of saturated fat per day. Remember that fat is linked to heart disease and cancer. Monounsaturated fats such as extra virgin olive oil, avocados, almonds, macadamia nuts and organic peanuts are good fats.
- Avoid red meat, pork and too much shellfish. They're high in cholesterol.
- Eat a high-fiber diet containing more than 20 grams of fiber a day. Most Americans get a third of that. A high-fiber diet will help prevent colon cancer and help eliminate toxins from the body.
- Strive for a low-sugar diet. Sugars are empty calories, and you don't need them. You can have a little, but practice moderation.

- Think low salt. Hide the salt shaker or switch to potassium salt.
- Avoid processed meats–they are also full of salt, and most contain nitrates.
- Avoid fermented fruits or vegetables. They are full of salt too, as are many sweets.
- Drink distilled water or reverse osmosis water.
- Take vitamins and minerals that include calcium, magnesium, beta carotene, vitamin E, vitamin C, vitamin D, cofactors, digestive enzymes, grape seed extract and coenzyme Q-10.
- Exercise. Options include brisk walking, calisthenics or weight lifting about three times a week.
- Pray fervently over your food. Bless your food at each meal.
- Pray in the Spirit, read the Word, meditate on the Scriptures and praise and worship daily since this ushers in the presence of God, which protects and covers us.

Notes

Chapter 5

The Colbert Plan for Optimal Health

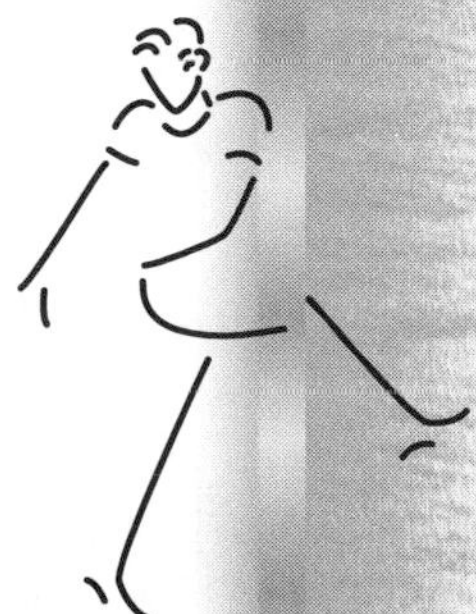

YOU WILL NOTICE SOME SURPRISING differences in your life when you begin to eat properly. You'll have much more energy, your mind will be sharper, and you will start losing weight. When you see the benefits you'll say, "I really don't want that fat, sugar and salt."

This diet will change your eating habits. People consuming large amounts of fat can go five to six

Living Healthy Tip No. 34

You should maintain good posture and practice deep breathing throughout the day. This will increase energy and may improve mental functioning.

hours between meals. This diet, however, lets you eat something about every three to four hours, because it includes midmorning and midafternoon snacks. The snacks help maintain your blood sugar level throughout the day so that you won't get that lightheaded feeling caused by swings in your blood sugar level.

BREAKFAST

You can have two power fruits: strawberries and tangerines.

- Orange juice: ½ cup
- Whole-grain cereal with strawberries and skim milk, or oatmeal with fructose
- Tangerine, soy protein drink and three macadamia nuts

Midmorning SNACK

- Fat-free yogurt with live culture
- Banana Fiber muffin (recipe on page 208)

LUNCH

You get two power vegetables and one power fruit.

- Tabouli with parsley and a small amount of olive oil
- Turkey sandwich with romaine lettuce, tomato and Dijon mustard on whole-grain bread
- Tangerine

Midafternoon SNACK *(around 3 P.M.)*

You can have any one of the following:

- Banana Fiber muffin
- Banana or another fruit
- Fat-free yogurt with live culture

DINNER

Try to have dinner before 7 P.M.

- Salad–the more colorful the better. Use your imagination with carrots, tomatoes, cucumbers, onions and mushrooms. Use a little red wine vinegar or one of the oils I've mentioned.
- One to two vegetables–broccoli is a wonderful vegetable, or you can have green beans, asparagus, cabbage or other low-starch vegetables
- Lean meat–chicken, fish or turkey
- Banana or fruit

Many people tend to eat a lot of carbohydrates at night. For those who want to lose weight, cut out your carbohydrates during this time. Carbohydrates include bread, rice, potatoes, pasta and corn. If these are favorites of yours, enjoy them at lunchtime or for a midmorning or midafternoon snack. Just don't eat them at night. Excess carbohydrates are converted to fat. In the evenings cut back your bread, rice, pasta and starchy vegetables. If you do, you'll see your weight begin to drop.

The Carbohydrate-Protein-Fat Plan

There is no perfect diet for everyone. A regimen that is healthy for one individual may actually be harmful to another due to food allergies, food sensitivities, gastrointestinal disturbances, blood types and other factors.

The diet of the majority of people in the United States contains excessive amounts of fat, sugar and salt, and it has a significant lack of fiber. The keys to the ultimate healthy lifestyle are found in eating primarily fruits, vegetables, whole grains, nuts, seeds, beans, legumes and lean meats. Avoid refined sugar and flour; avoid fats, which include hydrogenated fats, saturated fats and heat-processed polyunsaturated fats such as luncheon meats, cured meats, sausage and foods high in salt. Also limit your intake of red meat–choosing the leanest cuts possible.

The nutritional plan I recommend to my patients is the Carbohydrate-Protein-Fat Plan. Here's how it works. Each time you eat you should combine foods in a ratio of 40 percent carbohydrates, 30 percent proteins and 30 percent fats.

This program balances the correct ratio of carbohydrates, proteins and fats and controls insulin. Elevated insulin levels decrease physical performance and is one the primary predictors used in evaluating a person's risk of developing heart disease. To simplify this program, I will list the food categories and blocks, and then demonstrate how to use the blocks throughout the day. Let's look at some comparisons.

One block of protein is equal to 7 grams of protein, which is equivalent to approximately 1 oz. of meat such as beef, chicken breast or turkey breast.

One block of carbohydrates is equal to 9 grams of carbohydrates, which is equivalent to ½ slice of bread, ¼ bagel, ⅕ cup of rice, ⅓ banana, ½ apple or ¼ cup of pasta. This will be explained in greater detail later.

One block of fat is equal to 1.5 grams of fat, which is equivalent to ⅓ teaspoon of olive oil, six peanuts, three almonds or 1 tablespoon of avocado.

You will be getting much larger portion sizes than each individual food block. In fact, the average sedentary woman will get three food blocks at each meal, one food block midmorning, one food block midafternoon, and one food block at bedtime. An active female, who exercises three to four times a week for at least thirty minutes, may have four food blocks with each meal and one food block between meals and at bedtime.

A sedentary male may have four food blocks at each meal and one food block between meals and at bedtime, whereas the active male, who exercises three to four times a week, may have five or six food blocks at each meal and one food block between meals and at bedtime.

Let's discuss the different food blocks–starting with carbohydrate.

Carbohydrate Blocks

Fruit

- 1 tangerine, lemon, lime, kiwi or peach
- ½ apple, orange, grapefruit, pear or nectarine

- ⅓ banana, 1 cup strawberries or raspberries
- ¾ cup cubed watermelon or cubed cantaloupe
- ½ cup cubed honeydew melon, cherries, blackberries, blueberries, grapes, cubed pineapples or papaya
- ⅓ cup applesauce or mango

Juice

- ¼ cup grape or pineapple
- ⅓ cup apple, grapefruit, orange or lemon
- ¾ cup V8 juice

Cooked vegetables

- ⅛ cup baked beans
- ⅕ cup sweet potatoes or mashed potatoes
- ¼ cup lentils, kidney beans, black beans, red beans, lima beans, pinto beans, refried beans or corn
- ⅓ cup peas or baked potato
- 1 cup asparagus, green beans or carrots
- 1¼ cup broccoli, spinach or squash
- 1⅓ cup cabbage
- 1½ cup zucchini, Brussels sprouts or eggplant

- 1¾ cup turnip greens
- 2 cups cauliflower, collard greens

Raw vegetables

- 1 cucumber
- 2 tomatoes
- 1 cup onions (chopped), snow peas
- 1½ cup broccoli
- 2 cups cauliflower
- 2½ cups celery, green peppers (chopped)
- 3 cups cabbage, mushrooms (chopped)
- 4 cups romaine lettuce (chopped), cucumber (sliced)
- 6 cups spinach

Grains

- ⅕ ounces brown or white rice
- ¼ cup cooked pasta
- ⅓ cup cooked oatmeal (or ½ ounce dry), or grits
- ¼ bagel or English muffin
- ½ biscuit, waffle, or ½ of a 4-inch pancake, flour tortilla
- ½ ounce dry cereal

- 1 rice cake or corn tortilla
- 4 saltine crackers

High sugar items

- ½ tablespoon honey or molasses
- 2 tablespoons maple syrup
- 2 tablespoons ketchup, jelly (choose fructose jelly)

Protein Blocks

Meats

One ounce of skinless chicken breast, skinless turkey breast or free-range chicken. Or 1 ounce of skinless dark meat of turkey, skinless dark meat of chicken, hamburger with less than 10 percent fat, lean pork chop, lean ham, lean Canadian bacon, lean lamb or veal.

Note: I do not recommend eating pork and ham regularly. If an individual has a degenerative disease, he or she should avoid these meats completely.

Fish

Eat 1½ ounces of the following: salmon, mackerel, orange roughy, red snapper, sole, mahi-mahi, trout, halibut or grouper.

Eggs, dairy products and soy protein

Eggs—one whole egg or three egg whites; dairy products—1 ounce low-fat cheese, ¼ cup low-fat cottage cheese; soy protein—⅓ ounce of protein powder, ¼ soy burger, three ounces of tofu

Fat Blocks

- ⅓ teaspoon almond butter, olive oil, canola oil or flaxseed oil
- ½ teaspoon natural peanut butter
- 1 teaspoon olive oil and vinegar dressing, light mayonnaise or chopped walnuts
- 1 tablespoon avocado, guacamole
- 1 whole macadamia nut
- 1½ teaspoons almond (slivered)
- 3 almonds, olives, pistachios, cashews
- 6 peanuts

My Recommendations

For a woman, I recommend three to four blocks per meal with one food block between meals–midmorning, midafternoon and before bedtime. For a man I suggest four to six food blocks per meal, with one to two blocks midmorning, midafternoon and before bedtime. Men with a greater level of physical activity should have between five to six food blocks usually with each meal. Men who are sedentary should only have four. The same principle applies to women. Those who are sedentary should have only three food blocks per meal, and active women should have approximately four blocks.

As an example, four food blocks per meal is 4 ounces of chicken–for your four protein blocks; 1 cup of cooked asparagus, one head of lettuce and 1½ cups of red beans for your four carbohydrate blocks; and olive oil and vinegar dressing (1½ tablespoons) as your four fat blocks.

To simplify this meal plan even more, picture the palm of your hand; imagine placing a piece of protein (such as a piece of chicken, turkey, fish or lean red meat) the size of your palm. Next cup your hands and picture putting in the amount of vegetables or fruit that you can hold. You should then add one of the following: twelve almonds, twelve cashews (or pistachio nuts) or twenty-four peanuts. You are holding the ingredients for your healthy meal.

It's best to limit starches dramatically, which include bread, bagels, crackers, pasta, rice, pretzels, popcorn, beans, cereals, corn, potatoes, potato chips, corn chips and any other starchy item. I recommend "grazing" through the day–eating a fairly large breakfast, lunch and dinner and smaller midmorning, midafternoon and evening snacks. Eat the evening meal before 7 P.M. and take the evening snack preferably before 9 P.M.

People who have degenerative diseases such as heart disease, high blood pressure, high cholesterol, diabetes, hypoglycemia, cancer or patients who desire optimal health, should follow the ultimate health recommendations along with the Carbohydrate-Protein-Fat plan.

The Basics

If the Carbohydrate-Protein-Fat plan is too complicated, simply follow these basic instructions:

1. Reduce the intake of high-starch foods, including bread, crackers, bagels, pretzels, corn, popcorn, potatoes, sweet potatoes, potato chips, pasta, rice, beans and bananas by one-half to three-fourths. Better yet, eliminate them all together.

2. Avoid all simple sugar foods such as candies, cookies, cakes, pies and donuts. If you must have sugar, use Sweet Balance, a sweetener made from kiwi fruit. Choose fruit instead of fruit juices.

3. Increase your intake of nonstarchy vegetables such as spinach, lettuce, cabbage, broccoli, asparagus, green beans and cauliflower.

4. Choose healthy meats such as turkey

breast, chicken breast, fish, free-range beef and low-fat cottage cheese. Select healthy fats such as nuts, seeds, flaxseed oil, extra virgin olive oil or small amounts of organic butter. Use extra virgin olive oil and vinegar as a salad dressing. Choose the healthy fats we have listed instead of polyunsaturated, saturated and hydrogenated fats.

5. Eat three meals a day consisting of fruit, nonstarchy vegetables, lean meat and good fat. You should also have a healthy midmorning, midafternoon and evening snack.

By following these guidelines I believe you will experience increased energy and improved health.

Banana Fiber Muffins

1 cup Fiber One cereal, crushed
1 cup mashed ripe banana (about 2 medium bananas)
⅔ cup fat-free plain or vanilla yogurt
½ cup pecans or walnuts
½ teaspoon vanilla
2 tablespoons olive oil
2 egg whites (or 1 egg)
1½ cups Bisquick Light
½ cup fructose
3 teaspoons baking powder
¼ teaspoon salt
½ teaspoons ground cinnamon, if desired

Heat oven to 400 degrees. Grease bottoms only of 10 medium muffin cups, 2½ x 1¼ inches. Mix cereal, yogurt, pecans (or walnuts) and vanilla in medium bowl. Let stand 5 minutes. Beat in oil and egg whites. Mix remaining ingredients; stir into cereal mixture just until moistened. Divide batter evenly among muffin cups. Bake 20 to 25 minutes or until light brown. Immediately remove from pan. Serve warm. Makes 10 muffins.

1 serving (1 muffin): 160 calories; protein, 4 gr; carbohydrate, 34 gr; fat, 3 gr; sodium, 210 mg; cholesterol, 0 mg; total dietary fiber, 5 gr.

Notes

Walking in Divine Health

A Final Word

It is important to remember that the nutrients in the foods we eat will determine our health and the quality of our life. Make sure that the foods you consume are nutritionally sound and that you follow God's laws for divine health.

As a physician I have been privileged to be present at many miracle crusades. Walking through the crowds, I've seen too many people whose bodies are broken down. These people are often overweight, many have been stricken with cancer, they suffer with arthritis pain in their knees, their backs are severely bowed with osteoporosis and the arteries leading to their hearts are full of plaque. It is suffering people like these who often come seeking a healing.

Many of these same people are touched by God miraculously, and they leave rejoicing at what the Lord has done for them. Yet scores of these sincere individuals return to their homes and go right back to their old habits–eating the same harmful foods. It is not really surprising that some of them develop the same diseases and conditions all over again. Some come back and say, "What's the matter? Why did God put this disease back on me?"

Now that you have read what I feel the Lord has inspired me to write, the choice is yours. I pray that you will choose a healthy lifestyle that will bring glory to God. I pray that like Moses, Joshua and Caleb, you will walk in divine health, and that even in your old age you will continue to be filled with energy, health and vigor.

Notes

Chapter 1: Stopping Cancer Before It Starts

1. Peter Greenwald, M.D., director of Division of Cancer Prevention and Control, National Cancer Institute; "Cancer Prevention Trials to Clarify Relationships Between Diet and Cancer," sponsored by AMA, NY, NY; 14 January 1993.

2. John Heinerman, Ph.D., *Dr. Heinerman's Encyclopedia of Nature's Vitamins and Minerals* (Paramus, NJ: Prentice Hall, 1998), 148.

Chapter 2: Slamming the Door on Heart Disease

1. "Coronary Artery Surgery Study: A Randomized Trial of Coronary Bypass Surgeries," Survival Data, Circulation. 68: 939-950, 1983.

2. George Mann, M.D., "Cardiovascular Disease in the Masai," *Journal of Arteriosclerosis Research* 4 (1964):239.

Chapter 3: Eating to Live

1. Paper presented at the Symposium on Environmental, Socioeconomic and Political Aspects of Pest Management Systems (Houston, TX: 1979). "Pest Control: Cultural and Environmental Aspects," David Pimentel and John Perkins (Boulder, CO: Westview Press for the American Association for the Advancement of Science, 1980).

2. *USA Today,* 15 March 1994.

Chapter 4: Finding Your Way Through the Vitamin and Supplement Maze

1. Weston A. Price, D.D.S., "Nutrition and Physical Degeneration," Price-Pottenger Nutrition Foundation, Inc., (1939).

2. D. Burkitt and H. Trowell, *Western Diseases: Their Emergence and Prevention.* (Cambridge, MA: Harvard University Press, 1981).

Don Colbert, M.D., was born in Tupelo, Mississippi. He attended Oral Roberts School of Medicine in Tulsa, Oklahoma, where he received a bachelor of science degree in biology in addition to his degree in medicine. Dr. Colbert completed his internship and residency with Florida Hospital in Orlando, Florida. He is board certified in family practice and has received extensive training in nutritional medicine.

If you would like more
information about natural and
divine healing, or information about
Divine Health Nutritional Products®,
you may contact
Dr. Colbert at:

DR. DON COLBERT

1908 Boothe Circle
Longwood, FL 32750
Telephone: 407-331-7007
(For ordering products only)

Dr. Colbert's website is
www.drcolbert.com.

Disclaimer: Dr. Colbert and the staff of Divine Health Wellness Center are prohibited from addressing a patient's medical condition by phone, facsimile or e-mail. Please refer questions related to your medical condition to your own primary care physician.

IF YOU ENJOYED

Walking in Divine Health,

here are some other titles from Siloam Press that can help you to live in health—body, mind and spirit . . .

A HEALTHY HEART
Francisco Contreras, M.D.
ISBN: 0-88419-765-4
Retail Price: $19.99

Even if you've never experienced heart problems, you need to read this book. In it noted oncologist Dr. Francisco Contreras shares his medical expertise and wisdom as he explains the causes and treatments for heart disease. You will learn why technology can't always help, and you'll discover powerful keys for reclaiming heart health.

BREAKING THE GRIP OF DANGEROUS EMOTIONS
Janet Maccaro, Ph.D., C.N.C.
ISBN: 0-88419-749-2
Retail Price: $19.99

Learn how to stop letting dangerous emotions rob you of your joy as you discover the truth about worry and stress. You can replenish your physical body with a cutting-edge nutritional program that will restore your health. Explore exciting and proven protocols for rebuilding and regenerating your body, mind and spirit.

INTIMACY
Douglas Weiss, Ph.D.
ISBN: 0-88419-767-0
Retail Price: $21.99

Revitalize and recapture the excitement and joy that you once felt with your mate with this one-hundred-day program. Let Douglas Weiss, Ph.D., a licensed professional counselor and the executive director of Heart to Heart Counseling Centers, teach you how to energize your relationship and create spiritual, emotional and physical closeness. Learn to identify destructive emotional roadblocks, how to discuss your sexual desires, how to connect emotionally and how to let go of the past.

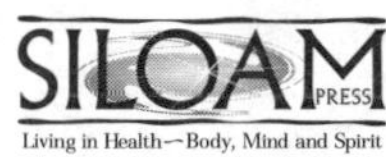

To pick up a copy of these titles, contact your local Christian bookstore or order online at www.charismawarehouse.com.